SARAH FIT

—GET—

SKINNY

AGAIN!

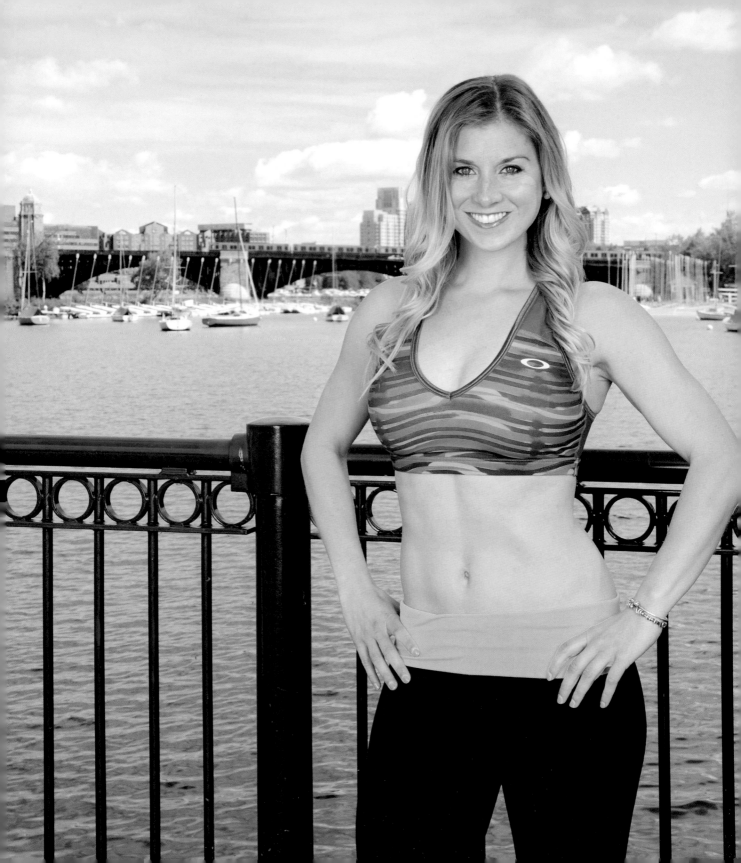

SARAH FIT

—GET—

SKINNY

AGAIN!

+ THE RIGHT EXERCISES TO +
GET BACK YOUR DREAM BODY
AND THE SECRETS TO
LIVING A FIT LIFE

SARAH DUSSAULT
YOUTUBE FITNESS STAR

PAGE STREET
PUBLISHING CO.

PAGE STREET
PUBLISHING CO.

First published in 2013 by
Page Street Publishing Co.
27 Congress Street, Suite 103
Salem, MA 01970
www.pagestreetpublishing.com

Distributed by Macmillan; sales in Canada by The Canadian Manda Group; distribution in Canada by The Jaguar Book Group.

16   15   14   13   1   2   3   4   5

ISBN-13: 978-1-62414-032-7
ISBN-10: 1-62414-032-7

Library of Congress Control Number: 2013942410

Cover and book design by Page Street Publishing Co.
Photography by Matthew Modoono Photography

Printed and bound in China

Page Street is proud to be a member of 1% for the Planet. Members donate one percent of their sales to one or more of the over 1,500 environmental and sustainability charities across the globe who participate in this program.

+ AS CLICHÉD AS IT MAY BE, THIS BOOK IS DEDICATED 100% TO MY BLOG READERS

AND YOUTUBE VIEWERS. WITHOUT YOU, I LITERALLY WOULD NOT BE A PUBLISHED AUTHOR.

I'M AMAZED BY YOUR DETERMINATION AND DEDICATION EVERY DAY. I FEEL BLESSED TO

HAVE BEEN GIVEN THE OPPORTUNITY TO HELP CHANGE YOUR LIVES AND MAYBE MAKE THE

WORLD A LITTLE BIT HEALTHIER, ONE FAN AT A TIME. I DO READ ALMOST EVERY SINGLE

COMMENT. YOUR INPUT HAS SHAPED THE DIRECTION OF MY CAREER,

AND I HOPE I DO NOT DISAPPOINT YOU WITH MY FIRST BOOK. +

CONTENTS

Introduction: To The 99% Who Are Not Naturally Skinny   9

PART ONE: TIME TO GET ON YOUR FITNESS

CHAPTER 1:

TIME TO SWEAT AT HOME   17
MY FAVORITE EXERCISES YOU CAN DO AT HOME WITH MINIMAL TO
NO EQUIPMENT THAT WILL PRODUCE THE BEST BURN

CHAPTER 2:

TIME TO HIT THE GYM   73
MY MOST EFFECTIVE ROUTINES AND EXERCISES USING THE BEST MACHINES

CHAPTER 3:

TIME TO SPARE 10 MINUTES   111
WHAT TO DO WHEN YOU ONLY HAVE 10 MINUTES AND SPECIFIC GOALS IN MIND

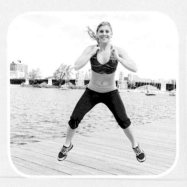
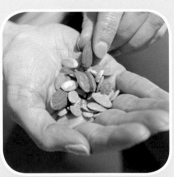
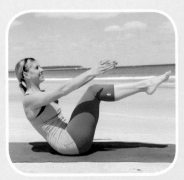

PART TWO: TIME TO EAT CLEAN TO GET LEAN

CHAPTER 4:

TIME TO EAT RIGHT 155
FRESH, FIT & SIMPLE RECIPES WITH REASONABLY PRICED INGREDIENTS

CHAPTER 5:

TIME TO DETOX 189
THE PROS AND CONS OF CLEANSES AND DIETS AND HOW TO TRY ONE SAFELY

CHAPTER 6:

TIME TO BE SOCIAL 195
MY TRIED AND TRUE TIPS FOR EATING HEALTHFULLY AT RESTAURANTS AND
DRINKING AT PARTIES WITHOUT BEING AWKWARD

PART THREE: TIME TO LIVE THE FIT LIFE

CHAPTER 7:

TIME TO GET SKINNY AGAIN 207
FAIL TO PLAN, PLAN TO FAIL. CREATING A ROADMAP TO SUCCESS

CHAPTER 8:

MY STORY 211
HOW I DISCOVERED MY PASSION FOR HEALTH AND FITNESS AND BUILT IT INTO
AN EMPIRE, AND HOW YOU CAN, TOO

Resources	215
Acknowledgments	216
About the Author	219
Index	220

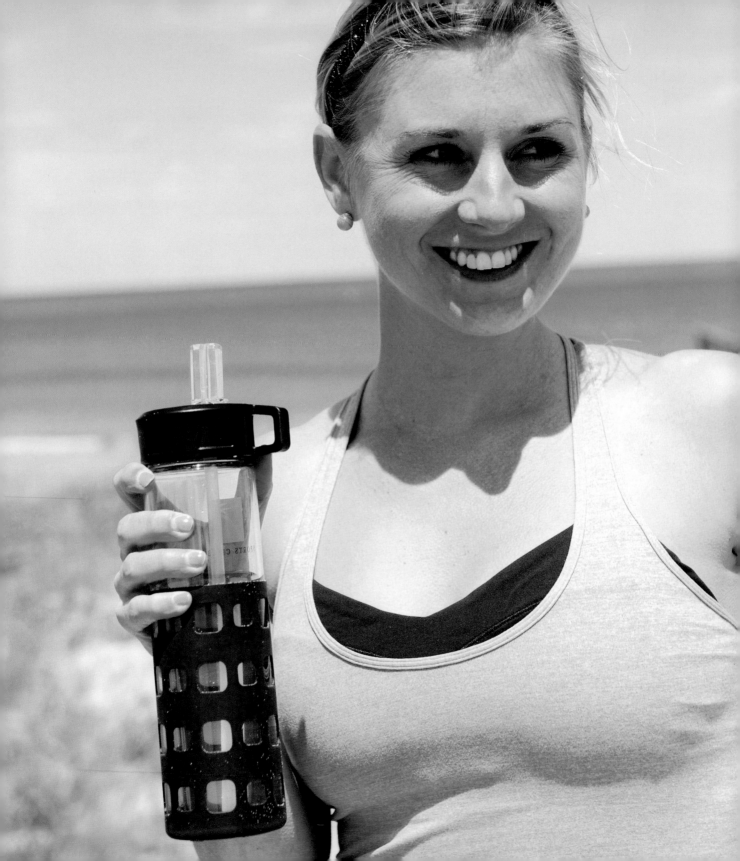

TO THE 99% WHO ARE NOT NATURALLY SKINNY

I've been training people on YouTube since 2006. With over 120 million lifetime views, I'm proud to have helped inspire and change many lives. I started making videos because I wanted people to have free access to good workouts that would help them lose weight and get healthy. I wanted to spread the truth that exercise is a cheaper alternative to many medications. My goal was to create something that I once needed. I wanted to pay it forward.

I'm not naturally skinny. I love to work out, but I also have a life and love to eat. I love dessert, cocktails and nachos. After a few too many late-night pizzas in college, I started to read most of the diet books that were out at the time, but the recipes had too many ingredients and were too time consuming and expensive! The workouts usually seemed to be geared toward beginners or people who had much more weight to lose than I did, and they were always limited in terms of where I could do them. I needed a resource that had workouts I could do in my dorm room, at the gym or outside depending on my schedule and mood.

I wanted to create a book that solved all these dilemmas, but I also wanted to create a program that you would want to follow, that you would read and think, *I can lose weight without sacrificing my social life? I can lose weight without hiring a personal trainer?* My methods are simple, easy to remember and affordable when it comes to getting back the body you feel proud to show off.

I wrote this book for the women out there like me who had a coach or parent dictating their workouts and meals up until or through college. Or perhaps you never played sports in school but were always naturally skinny and, all of sudden, in your twenties or thirties you've noticed your body has slowly begun to put on weight. As we get older our metabolisms slow down and we have more social opportunities that involve lots of empty calories. Studies have shown that when you move in with a boyfriend or become a newlywed, you are likely to gain weight. And if you have a desk job with long hours, the odds are stacking up against you. It seems that we are doomed, but I am here to tell you that we are not.

I want you to feel sexy and confident again. I'm going to show you my favorite moves that will sculpt and lift your cute little butt. I'm going to teach you the sweaty interval workouts I love that helped me melt five pounds of fat off my body while traveling for work in Hawaii. I'll list for you the ingredients to keep on hand so you can make nutritious, simple and delicious meals.

I didn't earn over 100,000 YouTube subscribers overnight. It took deliberate effort and hard work. Similarly, losing weight doesn't happen by accident. Viewers noticed changes in their own bodies after following my videos and kept coming back for more. Now I'm sharing my plan with you so you don't have to watch another YouTube video ad while waiting for the good stuff!

Whether you are in college, a new graduate or a seasoned working woman, this book is going to show you what it's like to get in shape, lose the unwanted weight, boost your confidence and feel healthy! It's not about getting skinny again for vanity, it's about feeling good about the way you look, and maintaining your health for a long and prosperous life!

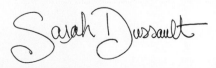

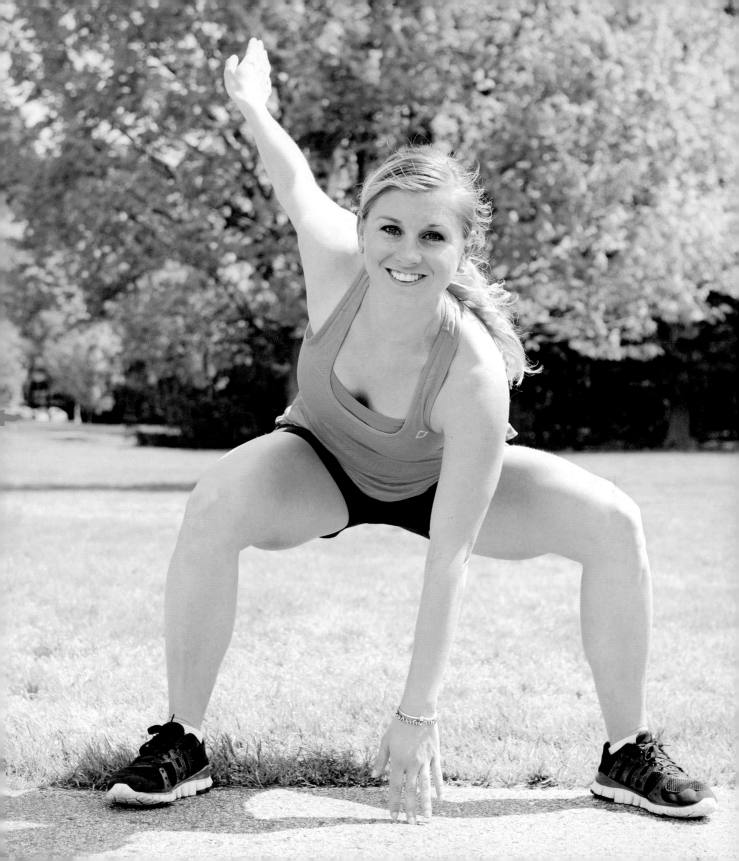

PART ONE

TIME TO GET ON YOUR FITNESS

CREATING A FITNESS SCHEDULE

I'm pretty sure that I'm in the minority, but I love working out. I didn't always, however, love what now brings me joy. In high school I never thought twice about working out. I had soccer and track. Practices, meets and games were my exercise. I had to train during the summer for soccer tryouts and running a timed 1.5 miles/2.4 km seemed like a marathon.

In between seasons I would go to the gym to stay in shape. I remember hopping onto an elliptical next to the 20-something assistant track coach one day. I stopped after 15 minutes, but she continued for at least 30. "Oh, my gosh! How long are you going to do that thing for? Aren't you bored?" I asked.

She responded, "One day, you'll understand." A few years later, I did.

Whether or not you played sports in high school or college, you most likely were never given a schedule for what a fitness routine should look like for your physical well-being. That aside, what should it look like to get skinny again?

Exercise is a science and the recommendations are always changing. Currently, it is advised to get least 150 minutes of moderate cardiovascular exercise each week. This can be achieved through 30 to 60 minutes of moderate activity 5 days a week or 20 to 60 minutes of vigorous activity 3 days a week. You can break this up as well into increments of 10 minutes.

In addition, 2 to 3 days a week, adults should train most muscle groups through resistance exercises. Flexibility training 2 to 3 days a week is also recommended. I hope I didn't I lose you there with all the numbers, but the rest of the book is going to be very simple. I promise!

SO HOW SHOULD YOU APPLY THESE RECOMMENDATIONS USING WHAT IS IN THIS BOOK?

First, I want you to create a plan. If you make a schedule for yourself and put it in your calendar you will be more likely to stick to it. One of my favorite expressions is "Fail to plan, plan to fail." It is so true. When I have an appointment to work out with a trainer, I never miss it. In your calendar I want you to write out exactly what you plan to do each day and designate a time. If something comes up, you can always shuffle things around, but don't cancel on your workouts. This is why people who exercise in the morning tend to do it more regularly and are less likely to skip out.

To get skinny again and lose those stubborn pounds, I have found that my clients and I have the most success with 3 days of cardio and 2 to 3 days of strength training. I also love yoga, but finding time to fit that in depends on your fitness personality.

YOUR FITNESS PERSONALITY

Gym Rat: You love your gym. You hate to exercise at home. You can use this entire book for your workouts. The at-home portion just does not include equipment. You can still do it at the gym on the floor or in an empty group exercise room.

Gym-Free Frugalista: You love saving money and work out often at home with DVD's or free YouTube workouts. If you own zero gym equipment, stick to the at-home part of this book. You'll be all set to get skinny with just this portion. If you own a pair of dumbbells, exercise ball and resistance band, you will be able to do most of the gym workouts as well. Feel free to try them at home also.

Exercise Enthusiast: You have a gym membership, but you also like to work out at home when you can't get there. Go ahead, mix and match the workouts from the gym and at-home chapter.

FITNESS SCHEDULE

DAY 1:	Strength training
DAY 2:	Cardiovascular
DAY 3:	Strength training
DAY 4:	Cardiovascular
DAY 5:	Strength training/stretching
DAY 6:	Longer than usual workout: Cardio
DAY 7:	Active rest/stretch

HOW MANY DAYS A WEEK SHOULD I WORK OUT?

Ideally, aim to work out 5 to 6 days a week to see optimal results using my program. Remember, losing weight is hard and takes time and commitment.

The Time to Get Skinny Again program is based on working out 6 days a week. If you want you can combine 2 days to give yourself an extra day off, but give yourself at least 1 day of rest between strength-training sessions. Depending on how much time you have and your access to a gym, there are a variety of options for you to choose from in this book.

Losing weight is 85% diet. If you do not have time to work out and your only goal is to lose weight, you really do not need to do the workouts. Seriously. You won't get skinny again quickly or be able to show off a chiseled stomach, but you will eventually lose weight.

There are many studies that have shown working out for as little as 10 minutes helps relieve stress, reduces depression, improves your memory, builds self-esteem, boosts self-confidence, releases endorphins that make you feel happy immediately, improves brain function, and may help prevent numerous diseases and cancers. I know you bought this book to lose weight, but there are so many more amazing benefits to sweating it out.

If you can't find time to exercise, just focus on your diet and making smart decisions about what foods you put in your mouth.

WHERE DO YOU FIT IN THE STRETCHING?

Feel free to add in as much stretching as you like. Many of the workouts have warm-ups built into them, but it is up to you to stretch afterward as part of a cooldown to prevent muscle soreness. I highly recommend the foam-rolling sequence found in chapter 2 after the strength-training routines if time permits. If you are interested in purchasing one to have at home, a foam roller costs between $10 and $40. Otherwise, the yoga stretch sequence in chapter 1 will help alleviate soreness. You have the option to do either routine after your workouts, or on Day 7 on its own as part of your active rest day. Make sure to fit in at least 2 stretching sessions a week.

HOW LONG DO I REALLY NEED TO WORK OUT?

For most of the workouts in the Time to Get Skinny Again program, you will be working out for 30 to 60 minutes at a time.

If you do not have time to fit in an entire workout, chapter 3 is dedicated to 10-minute workouts. The shorter workouts tend to be more intense, and for a reason. Try to squeeze in 1 or 2 first thing in the morning before jumping in the shower to start your day. If it's a cardio day, do the routine under "Goal: Lose Weight"; otherwise, pick one of your favorite toning routines.

For Day 6, you are encouraged to work out up to 50% longer than your typical cardio workout. This means that if you usually go running for 40 minutes, aim for 60 minutes.

DO I HAVE TO START DAY 1 ON A MONDAY?

The answer is no. You can start Day 1 on a Wednesday if you want. Rather than choose a random day to start, however, decide which day you want to *rest*. If you know you enjoy Saturday for shopping and watching movies, Day 7 should be a Saturday, which would make Sunday Day 1.

In this book I encourage you to take classes at your gym or local studio if that is something you enjoy. If you love a specific class or teacher, work that into your schedule. For example, if your favorite instructor teaches a fabulous 60-minute spin class that you and your friends always go to on Thursday morning, make sure that Day 2, 4, or 6 (also known as your cardio days) falls on Thursday.

M	T	W	TH	F	SA	SU
At Home Strength #2	Outdoor Cardio #3	At Gym Strength #1	Spin Class 60 mins	30 min Yoga 10-min Abs 10-min Butt	60 min RUN!	REST
At Gym Strength	At Gym Cardio	Barre Bootcamp at My Gym	Outdoor Cardio #2	At Home Strength #2	90 min Yoga	REST

If you have a gym membership but enjoy working out on your own as well, you have the most options. You can go to a class or follow one of the at-home workouts or one meant to be done at the gym. Mix it up. Keep it interesting and accessible.

If you do not have a gym membership, you can still do the gym workouts but will need to invest in a few pieces of equipment, such as a pair of dumbbells and a physioball, each of which costs between $15 and $35. There are alternative moves suggested for the few exercises that use a different piece of equipment.

If you follow my plan, these workouts will help you lose weight and get skinny again.

Are you ready to see your workouts?

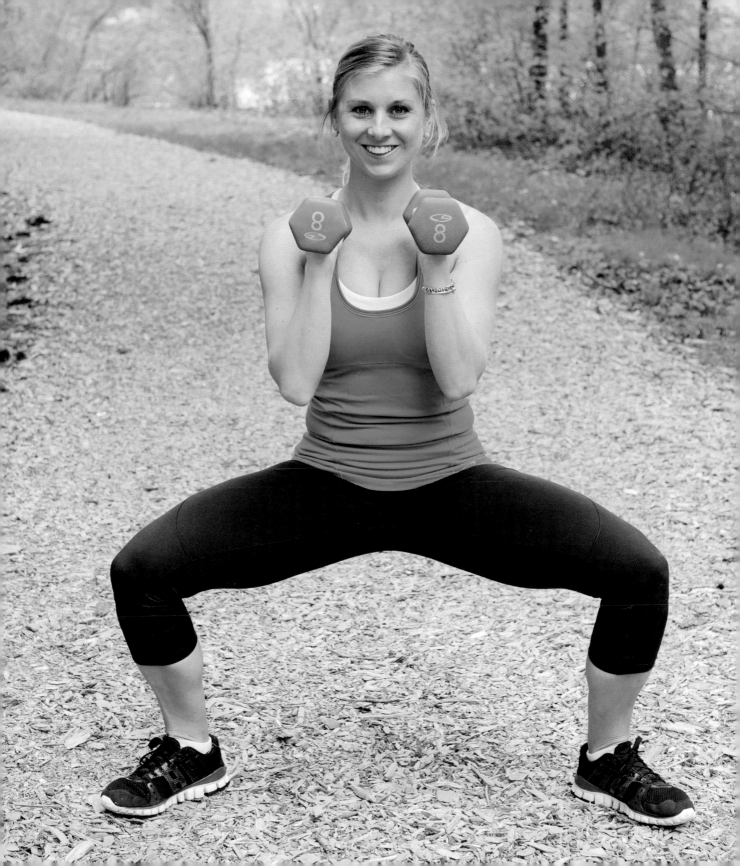

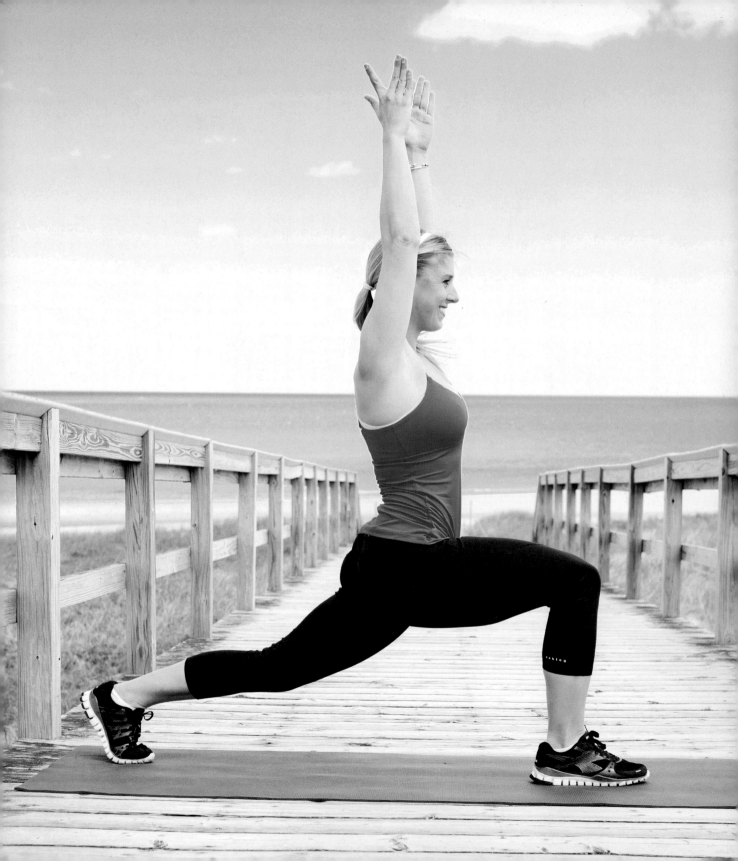

CHAPTER 1

TIME TO SWEAT AT HOME

The beauty of working out in the comfort of your own home is feeling judgment-free and having schedule flexibility. You don't have to commute to any studio or check to see if it is still open at night. You also don't have to wait to use any equipment, which makes it potentially the most efficient workout environment.

If time or money is tight, home workouts may be your best bet to getting skinny again. If you travel a lot, being able to sweat on your own without fancy equipment will also be your saving grace when it comes to sticking to your workout schedule.

After my freshmen year of college I invested in a pair of dumbbells and found a perfect outdoor loop for running. After work I would come home and put on my workout clothes right away. Within an hour, I was running or using my weights on the deck. I successfully lost 15 pounds that summer.

In this chapter you will find my favorite exercises that you can do anywhere. Most of the moves require little or no equipment. They are safe and effective, and you don't have to worry about how you look while doing them!

SCHEDULE

DAY 1:	Strength	DAY 5:	Strength or yoga/stretch
DAY 2:	Cardiovascular	DAY 6:	Long day
DAY 3:	Strength	DAY 7:	Off
DAY 4:	Cardiovascular		

STRENGTH AT HOME

STRENGTH OPTION 1: BODY-WEIGHT TRI-SET

This workout is one of my absolute favorite ways to tone and sculpt my muscles while burning lots of calories. I do it sometimes even when I'm at the gym but you can do it anywhere.

Sometimes when you look at a workout on paper, you might feel unmotivated and overwhelmed by the number of exercises. This workout is made up of tri-sets. To combat any type of anxiety, write down the workout on a piece of paper and each time you complete a set, cross it off. You are completely done with those exercises and can move on to the next set of three. There's something about crossing off completed tasks that reinforces your goals.

A tri-set is made up of three moves that are meant to be done back-to-back without resting in between: this will keep your heart rate elevated and burn the maximum number of calories. After you have done each move once, rest for 30 to 45 seconds. Go back to the first exercise and repeat each one for a second set, again without resting between moves. Rest for 30–45 seconds as you transition to the next tri-set. Do each move as directed below. For all the exercises that isolate one side of the body, do all the reps on the same side before switching to the opposite.

TRI-SET 1

MOVE 1:	Plank, hold for 60 seconds
MOVE 2:	Single-Leg Hip Lifts, 20–30 lifts on each leg
MOVE 3:	Side Lunges, 12–15 lunges on each leg
Rest 30–45 seconds and repeat.	

TRI-SET 2

MOVE 4:	Single-Leg Squat Toe Raises, 12–15 reps on each leg
MOVE 5:	Reverse Plank with Leg Lifts, 30-second hold on each leg
MOVE 6:	Triceps Dips, 30 dips
Rest 30–45 seconds and repeat.	

TRI-SET 3

MOVE 7:	Y Supermans, 15 reps
MOVE 8:	Push-Ups, 25 push-ups, or until you can't do anymore
MOVE 9:	Side-Plank Reach Throughs, 12–15 reps on each side
Rest 30–45 seconds and repeat.	

MOVE 1: **PLANK**

Start with your hands on the ground directly below your shoulders, palms facing the ground and toes tucked under. Lift your hips off the ground to form a straight line from your shoulders to your ankles. Breathe out and pull your navel toward your spine as if someone were about to punch you in the stomach.

TIP: If you can't hold this for the full minute, start with 30 seconds. Need even more help? Hold for 5 to 10 seconds, rest for 5 seconds and hold again. Do this until you reach 30 seconds. This is one of the best moves you can do to flatten your stomach.

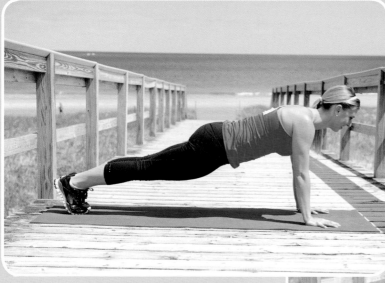

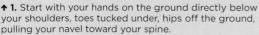
↑ **1.** Start with your hands on the ground directly below your shoulders, toes tucked under, hips off the ground, pulling your navel toward your spine.

↓ **BAD:** Don't slouch. Keep your spine straight from your shoulders to your ankles.

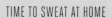

MOVE 2: **SINGLE-LEG HIP LIFTS**

Lie on your back, knees bent and fingertips grazing your seat. Lift one leg up straight toward the sky. Press through your heel on the ground and lift your butt up as high as you can, keeping your hips level and the extended leg still. Lower yourself and repeat. This move is going to lift your booty!

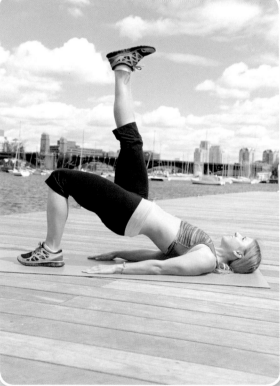

↓ **2.** Press through your heel on the ground and lift your butt up as high as you can, keeping your hips level and the extended leg still.

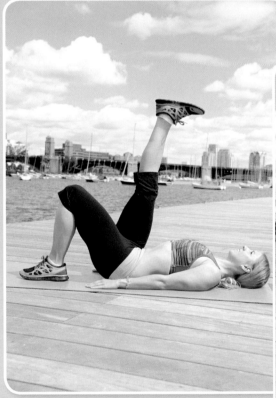

↑ **1.** Lie on your back with fingertips grazing your seat, one leg with the knee bent and foot on the ground and the other leg lifted straight toward the sky.

MOVE 3: **SIDE LUNGES**

Start with your feet hip width apart, standing tall, your fists in front of your chest. Step to the right, sinking down into a lunge on the right side, pushing your hips back so that your knee does not go beyond your toes. Your left leg should still be straight. Push off your right leg to return to the starting position. Finish all reps on the same leg before switching to the opposite. You're toning your inner thighs with this one.

TIP: Make sure your knee is in line with your toes when it bends. If your toes are facing forward but your knee is going out to the side, you are not doing the move correctly. Make sure both toe and knee are pointing in the same direction.

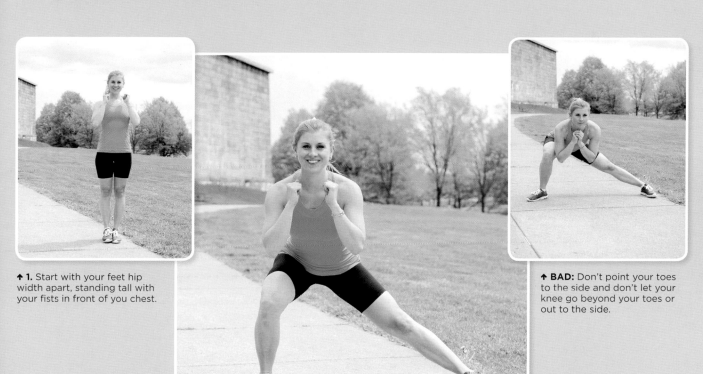

↑ **1.** Start with your feet hip width apart, standing tall with your fists in front of you chest.

↑ **BAD:** Don't point your toes to the side and don't let your knee go beyond your toes or out to the side.

↑ **2.** Step to the right, sinking down into a lunge on the right side.

MOVE 4: **SINGLE-LEG SQUAT TOE RAISES**

Begin by balancing on your left leg, your right leg slightly lifted off the ground in front of your body. Your hands are in fists in front of your chest. Slowly lower yourself into a squat position, keeping your right leg off the ground. When you are as low as possible, press through your left heel and return to a standing position. Lift up onto the ball of your right foot for a calf rise at the top before returning to the starting position. This is my favorite butt-shaping move!

TIP: When lowering into a squat, make sure your chest stays open and your core is engaged. Do not let your knee wobble to the right or left. Try to keep it steady and facing forward. Go slowly to start. To make this move more advanced, keep your lifted leg straight the entire time and lower yourself until your straight leg is parallel with the ground and your butt is nearly touching the ground.

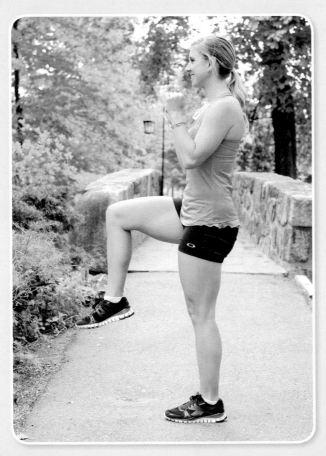

← 1. Balance on your left leg with your right leg slightly lifted off the ground in front of your body and hands in fists in front of your chest.

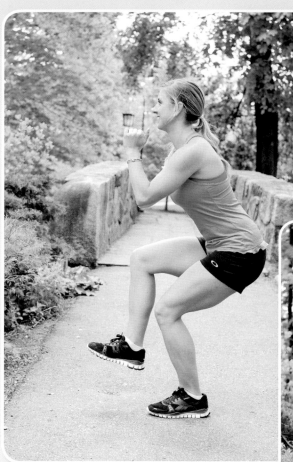

↑ 2. Slowly lower yourself into a squat position, keeping your right leg off the ground.

↓ 3. Lift up onto the ball of your left foot for a calf raise before returning to starting position.

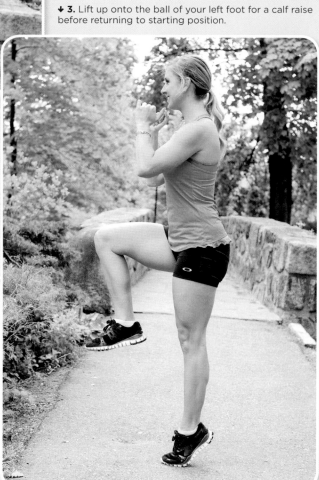

MOVE 5: **REVERSE PLANK WITH LEG LIFTS**

Sit on your butt with your hands by your sides. Your legs should be bent and your feet flat on the floor under your knees. Your fingers should be pointing toward your feet. Lift your hips up so that your torso and thighs are in a straight line, your glutes engaged. Lift your left leg up so that it forms a line from your chest to your ankle. Hold for 30 seconds. Lower your leg, rest for 20 seconds. Repeat, lifting your leg and holding for 30 seconds.

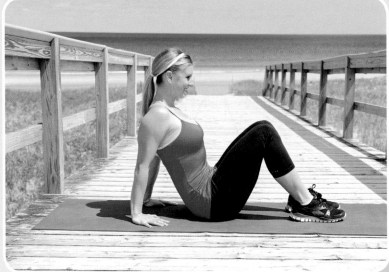

↓ 2. Lift your hips up so that your torso and thighs are a straight line and then lift your left leg up so that it forms a line from your chest to ankle. Hold for 30 seconds.

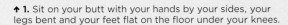

↑ 1. Sit on your butt with your hands by your sides, your legs bent and your feet flat on the floor under your knees.

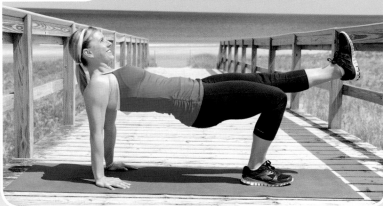

MOVE 6: TRICEPS DIPS

Sit with your butt on a bench or coffee table. Grab the edge of the table with both hands and push through the heels of your hands to lift your butt off the table. Slightly shift your hips forward a couple of inches. Keep your rib cage close to your biceps. Lower your hips toward the ground, bending at the elbows until they almost form a right angle. Press back up into starting position through the heels of your hands. This works your triceps for sexy tank top-ready arms.

TIP: The farther out your feet are from your hips, the more challenging this move will be. Try to keep your chest between your arms. Keep your butt close to the seat. If you don't have access to a bench, try this move on the ground.

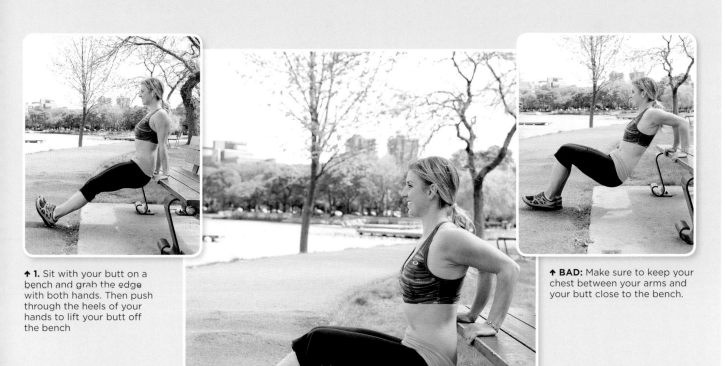

↑ **1.** Sit with your butt on a bench and grab the edge with both hands. Then push through the heels of your hands to lift your butt off the bench

↑ **BAD:** Make sure to keep your chest between your arms and your butt close to the bench.

↑ **2.** Slightly shift your hips forward a couple of inches and lower them toward the ground, bending at the elbows until you form an almost right angle.

MOVE 7: **Y SUPERMANS**

Lie down on the ground on your stomach with your arms reaching overhead in a Y position. Lift your head off the ground so that your nose just touches your mat. Engage your glutes. Breathe out as you lift your arms and torso up off the ground, engaging your core. Hold for a count of 1. Then return to starting position lowering arms back to the ground. This move helps improve your posture, so that you look leaner without even losing a pound!

TIP: Make sure to keep your shoulders pressed down, away from your ears, and squeeze shoulder blades together. Also engage your core and glutes during this exercise to protect your lower back.

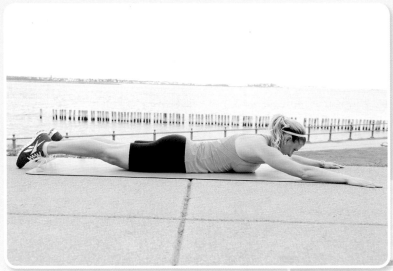

↓ **2.** Lift your heard, arms and torso off the ground, engaging your core. Hold for 1 count.

↑ **1.** Lie down on your stomach with your arms reaching overhead in a Y position.

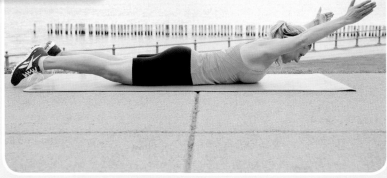

MOVE 8: **PUSH-UPS**

Starting position: Start in a high-plank position with your hands slightly wider than hip width apart. Your body should form a straight line from shoulders to ankles. Lower your body in a perfect line until your chest grazes the floor. Press back up to the starting position. This is a total-body power move that also helps get rid of upper-arm fat and creates a perky chest.

TIP: Make this move easier by dropping down to your knees, or by placing your hands on a wall or bench.

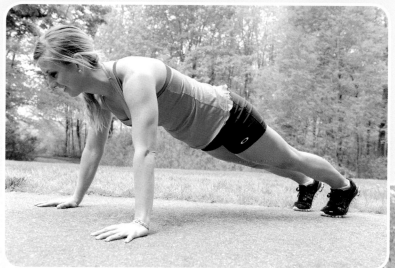

↓ 2. Lower your body in a perfect line until your chest grazes the floor. Then push back up to starting position.

↑ 1. Start in high-plank position with your hands slightly wider than hip width apart.

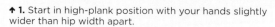

MOVE 9: SIDE-PLANK REACH THROUGHS

Starting position: Begin on your right side with your right hand underneath your right shoulder. Stack your left foot on top of your right foot. Lift your hips up so that your body forms a straight line from your shoulders to your ankles. Reach your left arm up toward the sky. Wrap your left hand around your midsection, as if you were giving yourself a single-arm hug. Rotate your left shoulder slightly toward the ground. Unwrap your arm and reach back up toward the sky. This move helps reduce those love handles for good!

TIP: If this is too hard, lower your right knee toward the ground.

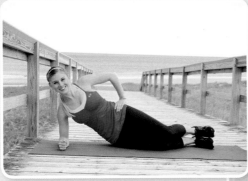

↑ **1.** Begin on your right side with your right hand underneath your right shoulder and your left foot stacked on top of your right foot.

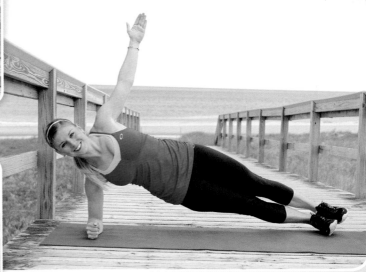

↑ **2.** Lift your hips up so that your body forms a straight line from your shoulders to your ankles while reaching your left arm toward the sky.

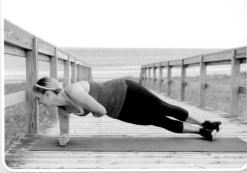

↑ **3.** Rotate your left shoulder slightly toward the ground. Then wrap your left hand around your midsection before reaching back toward the sky and going back to starting position.

STRENGTH OPTION 2: TIMED BODY-WEIGHT WORKOUT

This workout technically is categorized as being at-home accessible, but you can do it at the gym if you like. I love to sneak inside a group exercise studio to do my strength training in private. Many of these moves are perfect to do on hardwood floors with a towel, glider, or paper plate at home. If you don't have access to hardwood floors, I have included modifications.

I love this workout because not only does it hit every major muscle group but you can literally feel your muscles cinching together, getting tighter, stronger and more toned. While it may not be the highest calorie-burning workout in this book, it is a killer. The leg circles are an all-star move in my opinion. They are from a Pilates routine and helped me get my muscular legs (from high school soccer) toned and lean.

Do each exercise for 5 reps to warm up your body. When you feel ready to begin, grab a timer or your smart phone. Begin the stopwatch and do each move for the prescribed amount of reps, then move on to the next move without resting. Write down your time and rest for 1 or 2 minutes after you have completed all 9 moves. You are going to go through the sequence of moves 2 more times, for a total of 3 rounds. Aim to beat your previous time each round. Do this workout with a friend to make it a little competitive.

MOVE 1:	Inchworm Triceps Push-Ups, 10 reps
MOVE 2:	Side-Crunch V-sits, 20 reps
MOVE 3:	Sliding Reverse Lunges, 20 reps each leg
MOVE 4:	Sliding Side Lunges, 20 reps each leg
MOVE 5:	Leg Circles, 10 circles counterclockwise, 10 circles clockwise
MOVE 6:	Keg-Stand Shoulder Presses, 12 reps
MOVE 7:	Plank with Single Leg Lifts, lift each leg 30 seconds
MOVE 8:	Opposite-Arm and Leg Supermans, 10 reps
MOVE 9:	Kick-Downs, 12 reps

STRENGTH OPTION 2

MOVE 1: INCHWORM TRICEPS PUSH-UPS

Start by standing up tall, arms by your sides. Bend over at the hips to touch the ground. Slowly walk your hands out into a plank position. With your elbows close to your body, lower your body into a triceps push-up. Walk your feet in toward your hands and stand back up. This move works your core and upper body.

TIP: To make this move easier, lower your knees before performing the triceps push-up. Keep your legs as straight as possible throughout the exercise.

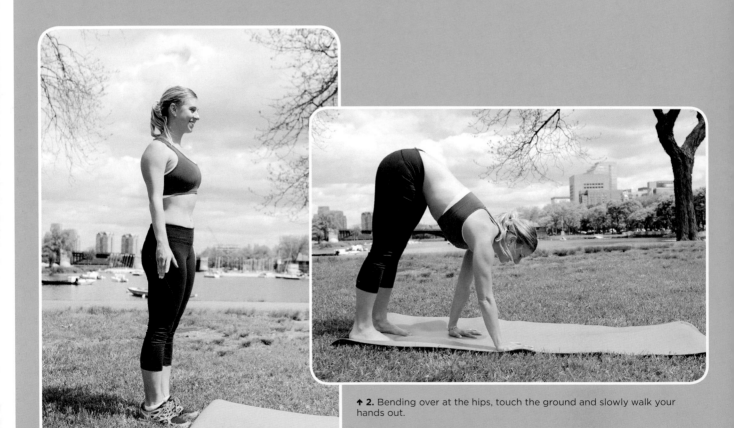

↑ 2. Bending over at the hips, touch the ground and slowly walk your hands out.

↑ 1. Start standing tall, arms by your sides.

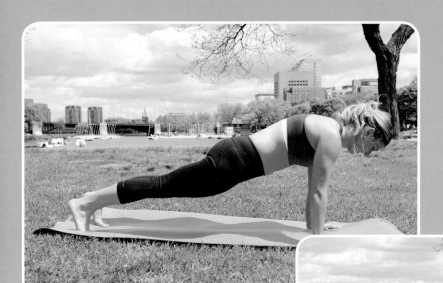

↑ 3. Walk your hands out until you are in a plank position.

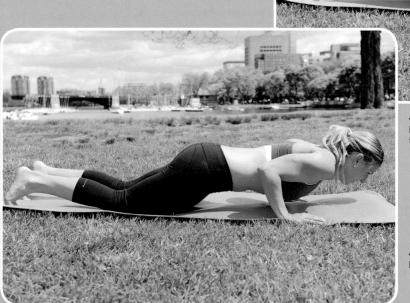

↑ 4. With your elbows close to your body, lower your body into a triceps push-up and then walk your feet in towards your hands and stand back up.

← BEGINNER: To make this move easier, lower your knees before performing the triceps push-up.

MOVE 2: SIDE-CRUNCH V-SITS

Sit on the ground, balancing on your tailbone with your legs together, your knees bent and feet up off the ground. Extend your legs out straight to the right as you lower your torso to the left. Crunch the right side of your obliques and return to the starting position as you exhale. This has been a staple in my routine since high school. It's helped me keep my tummy flat throughout the years!

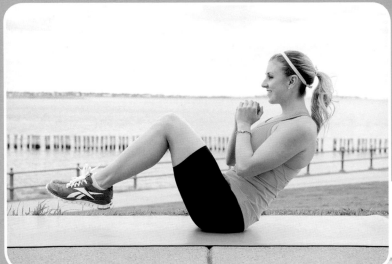

↑ **1.** Sit on the ground, balancing on your tailbone with your legs together, your knees bent and feet up off the ground.

↓ **2.** Extend your legs out straight to the right as you lower your torso to the left. Then crunch the right side of your obliques and return to start.

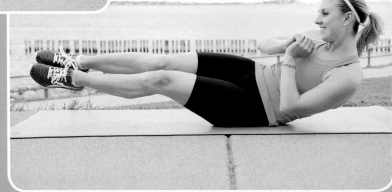

MOVE 3: SLIDING REVERSE LUNGES

Start with the ball of your left foot on top of a sliding accessory, such as towel or paper plate, or on a hard wooden surface, slightly behind your body. Position your feet about 4 inches/10 cm apart, your knees bent behind your toes in a stationary half squat. Quickly slide your left foot back behind your body, not lifting your left toes off of the sliding accessory. (If doing this move without a sliding accessory, hover working leg just above ground.) Glide your foot back until your left leg is straight while the right knee remains stationary. Quickly return to the starting position, still maintaining contact with the sliding accessory. Slide the left foot backward and forward for all 20 reps before switching to the opposite side.

TIP: The lower your beginning squat position, the more challenging this move will be. If you do not have hardwood or hard surface floors at home, try this move wearing socks on the carpet.

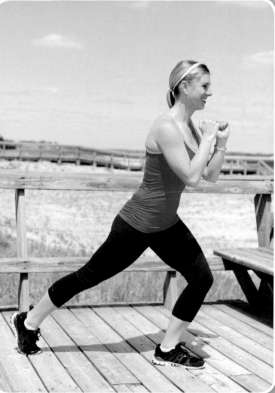

↓ **2.** Quickly slide your left foot behind your body, not lifting your left toes off the sliding accessory.

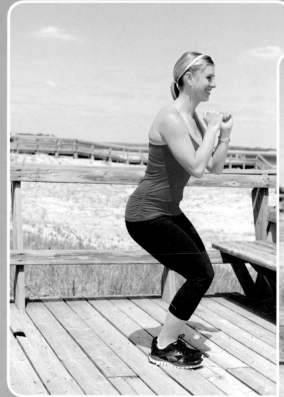

↑ **1.** Start with your feet about 4 inches apart and your knees bent behind your toes in a stationary half squat. Put the ball of your left foot on top of a sliding accessory, or do this exercise on a hard wooden surface.

MOVE 4: **SLIDING SIDE LUNGES**

Start in a half squat position with your right leg on a towel or other sliding accessory of choice. You can also do this move without an acessory by dragging your toes along the ground. Balance on your right leg. Extend your left leg out straight as far to the left as possible, dragging along the sliding accessory. Keeping your right leg stationary, still in a squat position, bring your left leg back to meet it. Repeat as quickly as possible. This move is working your inner thighs to help tone and slim them down.

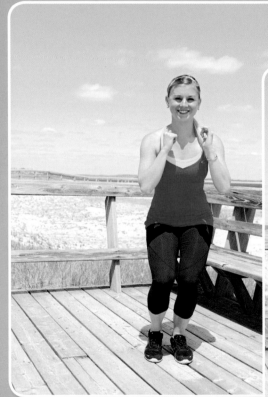

↑ **1.** Start in a half squat position with your right leg on a sliding accessory or hard wooden surface.

↓ **2.** Extend your right leg out straight as far to the left as possible.

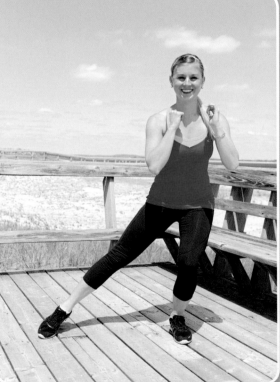

MOVE 5: **LEG CIRCLES**

Lie on your back with your left leg straight up toward the sky, toes pointed. Keep both hips glued to the ground. Draw an imaginary circle clockwise with your toes out and around your hips about the size of a large beach ball. After you draw 10 circles, go the opposite direction for 10 counterclockwise circles. Your movements should be slow and controlled.

TIP: Remember to keep your abs engaged and your hips on the ground.

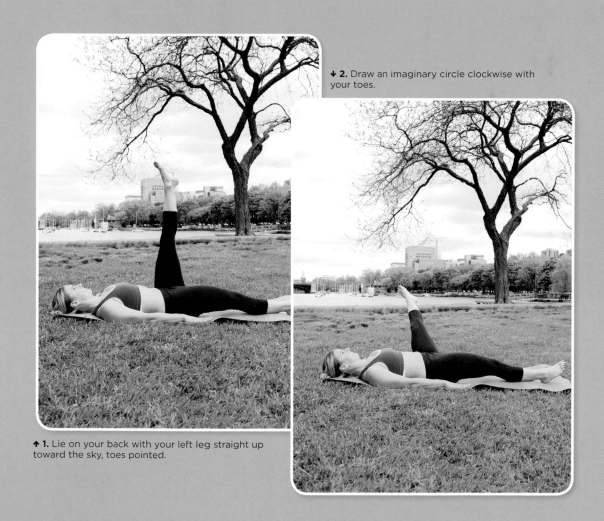

↓ **2.** Draw an imaginary circle clockwise with your toes.

↑ **1.** Lie on your back with your left leg straight up toward the sky, toes pointed.

MOVE 6: **KEG-STAND SHOULDER PRESSES**

Start in a low squat position with your hands out in front of you. Bend at the hips and lower your hands toward the ground, keeping your spine straight. Make contact with the ground, keeping your head between your biceps. Lower your head toward the ground as you bend and extend your elbows into a shoulder press. As you extend your arms, push off and return to the starting position. This move is sculpting your shoulders.

TIP: Keep your core engaged during this exercise for an added abs benefit. Make sure your shoulders stay away from your ears.

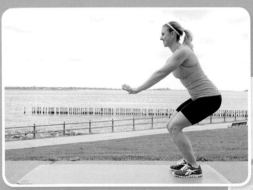

↑ **1.** Start in a low squat position with your arms out in front of you.

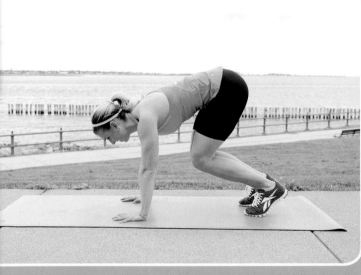

↑ **2.** Bend at the hips and lower your hands toward the ground, keeping your spine straight.

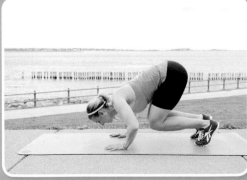

↑ **3.** Lower your head toward the ground as you bend your elbows into a shoulder press.

MOVE 7: PLANK WITH SINGLE-LEG LIFTS

Start by getting into a high plank position. Your body should be in a straight line from your shoulders to your ankles. Lift your left leg off the ground and hold for 30 seconds. Without resting, switch to lift your right leg and hold it up for 30 seconds. This move works not only your core but also your butt.

TIP: If this is too hard, alternate the leg lifts every 10 seconds. Take a 10-second break after holding a plank for 20 seconds. Repeat until you reach 1 minute. Make sure to keep your hips in line with your shoulders and ankles. Do not let them hike up or sink down if you get tired.

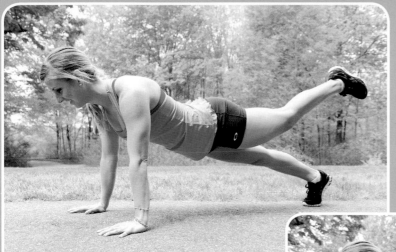

↑ **1.** Start by getting into a low plank position, and then lift your left leg off the ground and hold for 30 seconds. .

↓ **BAD:** Don't let your hips sink. Keep your spine straight and your core engaged.

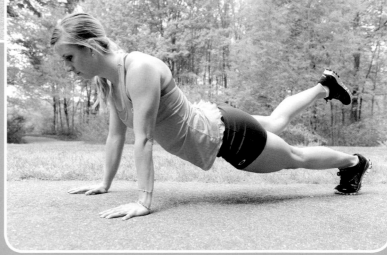

MOVE 8: **OPPOSITE-ARM-AND-LEG SUPERMANS**

Lie facedown on the ground with both arms extended over your head in a Y position. As you exhale, lift your right arm straight up a few inches off the floor as you lift your left leg a few inches up as well, squeezing the left glute. Hold for 1 count and then lower. Switch sides and repeat. This move is going to tone up your entire backside.

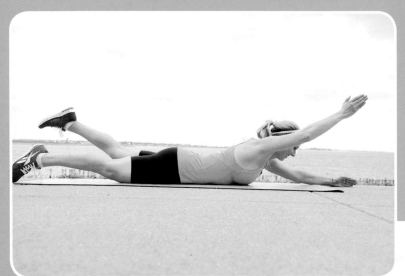

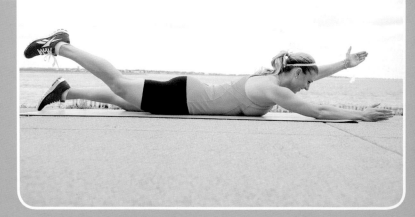

↓ 2. Lower your arm and leg and switch sides.

↑ 1. Lie facedown on the ground with both arms extended overheard in a Y position. Lift your right arm up a few inches as you also lift your left leg a few inches. Hold for 1 count.

MOVE 9: **KICK-DOWNS**

Lie down on your back with your hands underneath your buttocks and your feet extended straight up toward the sky. As you exhale, lower your legs as low as you can go before your lower back begins to pop up off the ground. Raise them back up to the starting position.

TIP: Lower your legs only as far as you comfortably can. Keep your navel pressed your into spine the entire time, as if someone were about to punch you in the gut.

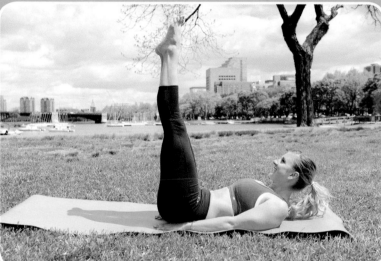

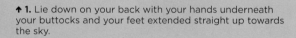

↑ **1.** Lie down on your back with your hands underneath your buttocks and your feet extended straight up towards the sky.

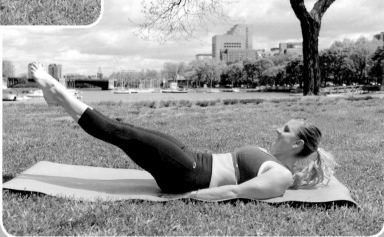

↓ **2.** Lower your legs as low as you can go before your lower back begins to pop off the ground.

CARDIO

When it comes to losing weight without dieting, cardio has been shown to produce the quickest results. For the most effective use of your time stick with interval training, in which you vary the intensity of your movements for specific periods. Studies have revealed that intervals burn more fat for fuel during a workout than steady-state cardio. It also makes your sweat session much less boring!

CARDIO OPTION 1: RAINY-DAY 20-MINUTE HIGH INTENSITY INTERVAL TRAINING (HIIT) WORKOUT

This workout is a series of 4-minute intervals featuring different cardio moves you can do at home. Most of the moves are quiet enough for you to do inside if you live in an apartment with neighbors below. This workout will take a total of 20 minutes to complete. Do each move at maximum intensity for 20 seconds. At the end of 20 seconds, you will get a 10-second rest. You will repeat this 20 seconds on, 10 seconds off, 8 times for a total of 4 minutes. By the end of each 4-minute interval, you should need a break. Go all-out for maximum results. You get a minute between sets in which you will be able to recover and catch your breath.

INTERVAL 1

MOVE 1:	Hover Jacks, maximum intensity for 20 seconds, rest 10 seconds
MOVE 2:	Jump Lunges, maximum intensity for 20 seconds, rest 10 seconds
MOVE 3:	Mountain Climbers, maximum intensity for 20 seconds, rest 10 seconds
MOVE 4:	Twisting Uprights, maximum intensity for 20 seconds, rest 10 seconds
Repeat Moves 1-4 including rest then take 1 minute break	

INTERVAL 2

MOVE 1:	Oblique Burpees, maximum intensity for 20 seconds, rest 10 seconds
MOVE 2:	Speed Skaters, maximum intensity for 20 seconds, rest 10 seconds
MOVE 3:	Froggers, maximum intensity for 20 seconds, rest 10 seconds
MOVE 4:	Speed Squats, maximum intensity for 20 seconds, rest 10 seconds
Repeat Moves 1-4 including rest then take 1 minute break	

INTERVAL 3

Same as interval 1

INTERVAL 4

Same as interval 2

CARDIO OPTION 1: INTERVAL 1

MOVE 1: **HOVER JACKS**

Start in high-plank position, your hands on the ground directly below your shoulders, palms facing the ground and toes tucked under. Your spine should be in a straight line from your neck to your tailbone. Squeeze your shoulder blades down away from your ears and toward each other. Gently bend your knees and jump so that your feet are wider than hip width apart. As soon as your toes hit the floor, jump so that your feet are back together, as if you were doing jumping jacks with just your lower body. Continue for 20 seconds, keeping your navel pulled in toward your spine and your back straight.

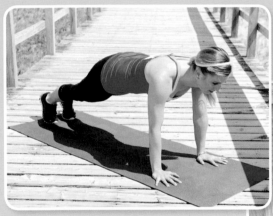

↑ **1.** Start in high-plank position.

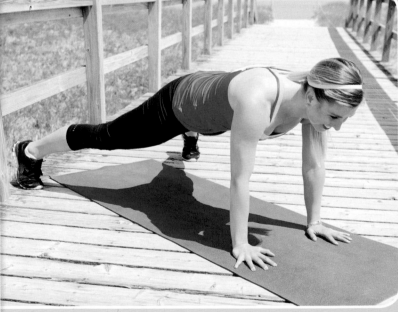

↑ **2.** Jump so that your feet are wider than hip width apart.

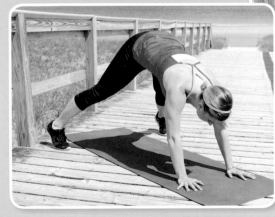

↑ **BAD:** Make sure to keep your spine in a straight line from your neck to your tailbone. Don't stick your butt up!

MOVE 2: JUMP LUNGES

Start in a gentle high-lunge position, that is, with your knees slightly bent, your right foot in front of the left, about 12 inches/30 cm apart. Lunge downward until your right thigh is parallel with the floor and left leg creates a right angle. Using your arms for momentum, press through your right heel and left toe to jump up and switch legs, lowering immediately back into another lunge. Do not let your front knee go past your toes, and make sure your back thigh is perpendicular to the floor as you lower your body. Make sure to land gently as well, to protect your knees. This move is going to burn fat while sculpting a killer lower body.

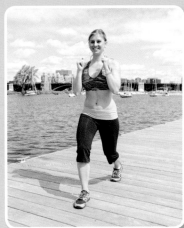

↑ **1.** Start in a gentle high-lunge position.

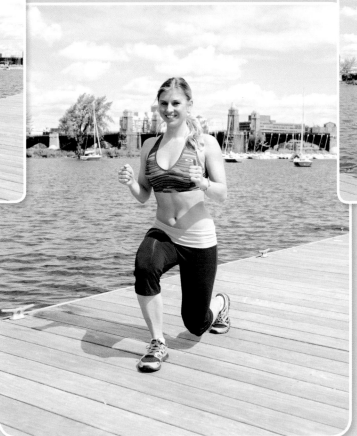

↑ **2.** Lunge downward.

↑ **3.** Jump up and switch legs, landing into another lunge.

MOVE 3: **MOUNTAIN CLIMBERS**

Start in high-plank position, feet shoulder distance apart, abdominal muscles engaged and spine in a straight line from neck to tailbone. Bring your right knee to your chest and hover over the ground. Quickly switch legs and bring your left knee to your chest as the right one fully extends. Continue to switch legs. If you are a beginner, you may bring your knees in one at a time slowly and skip the hang time, when both feet are off the ground at the same time. Not only does this move raise your heart rate, but it's also sculpting your abs.

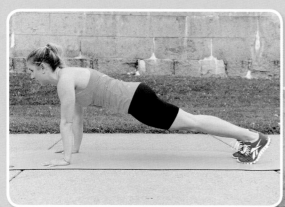

↑ **1.** Start in high-plank position.

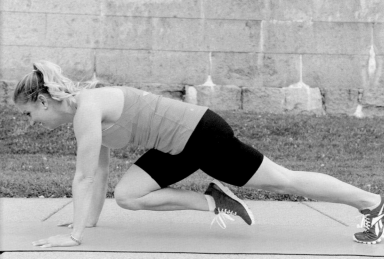

↑ **2.** Bring your right knee to your chest and then your left. Continue to switch legs.

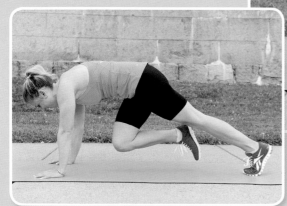

↑ **BAD:** Don't round your back. Keep your spine in a straight line from your neck to your tailbone.

MOVE 4: **TWISTING UPRIGHTS**

Start by standing tall with your arms out to your sides at shoulder height. Bend your arms at the elbow with your hands pointing up, simulating American football goalposts. Take a deep breath in and, as you exhale, raise your left knee as you bring your right elbow to meet it. Take a deep breath in as you return to the starting position, and bring your left elbow to your right knee as you exhale. Continue to alternate quickly as you twist at the waist. This is an amazing standing ab exercise, helping define your obliques.

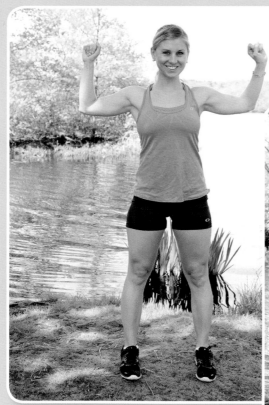

↑ 1. Stand tall with arms out to your sides at shoulder length and hands pointing up.

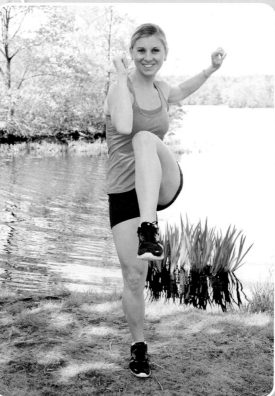

↓ 2. Bring your left knee to meet your right elbow and then switch.

MOVE 1: **OBLIQUE BURPEES**

Stand tall with hands reaching up toward the sky. Lower your hands to the ground and kick your feet out behind you. Rotate your right hip down toward the ground as you balance on the outside sole of your right foot and inner sole of your left foot. Your chin should be facing forward and your hands in a high plank position. You should feel this in your right obliques. (If you are a beginner, step one foot out at a time.) Quickly jump, feet in toward your hands, landing on the soles. Jump up tall, reaching for the sky. Repeat. If you would like a challenge, add a push-up at the bottom. Beginners can omit the jump. Get rid of your love handles with this exercise.

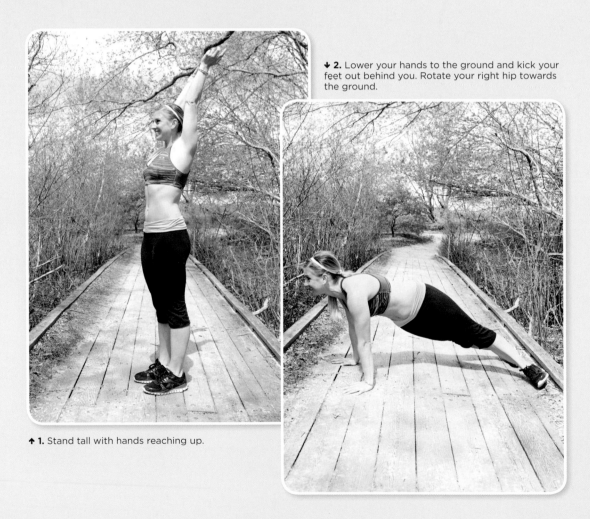

↓ **2.** Lower your hands to the ground and kick your feet out behind you. Rotate your right hip towards the ground.

↑ **1.** Stand tall with hands reaching up.

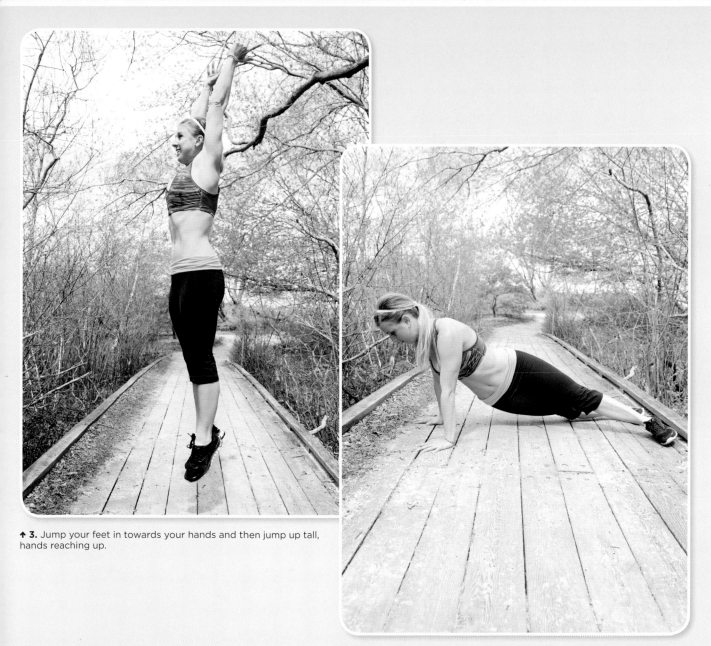

↑ **3.** Jump your feet in towards your hands and then jump up tall, hands reaching up.

↑ **BAD:** Don't slouch; keep your abs engaged and your spine straight.

MOVE 2: **SPEED SKATERS**

Start by balancing on your right leg, knee slightly bent. Your left leg is bent at the knee, your left foot slightly in front of your body. Keep your hands out in front for balance. Hop as far as you can to the left, landing gently on your left leg and lowering into a shallow single-leg squat. Push off your left leg and hop as far to the right as you can, gently landing on a slightly bent right leg. Repeat. You may use your arms naturally for balance and momentum. Keep your chin up, looking forward the entire time and keeping your back straight. Don't let your shoulders round forward. This is a booty-lifting special.

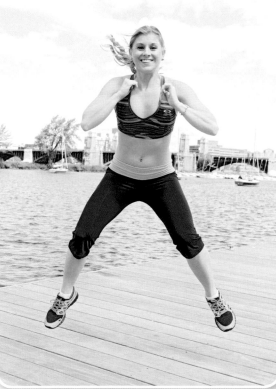

↓ **2.** Push off your right leg and hop as far as you can to your left, landing on a slightly bent left leg.

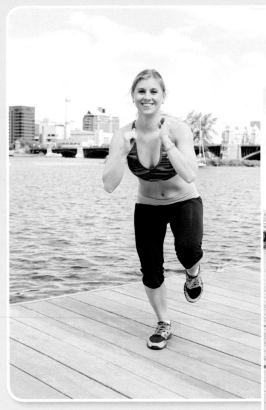

↑ **1.** Start by balancing on your right leg, knee slightly bent.

MOVE 3: **FROGGERS**

Start in high-plank position. Jump to bring your feet up toward your hands and slightly lift your hips. Land your feet to the outsides of your hands while keeping your core engaged. Keep your chin up and your eyes forward throughout the exercise. If you are a beginner, step your feet to the outside of your hands rather than jumping. Jump back into a high plank and repeat. Focus on using your core for a fat-blasting ab exercise.

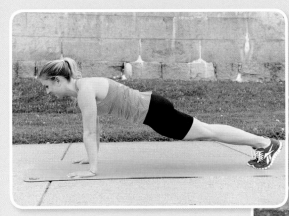

↑ **1.** Start in a high-plank position.

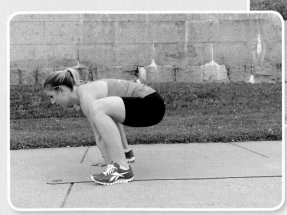

↑ **3.** Land your feet to the outsides of your hands.

↑ **2.** Jump to bring your feet toward your hands while lifting your hips.

MOVE 4: **SPEED SQUATS**

Start with your feet shoulder-width apart, standing up tall. Sit back onto your heels until your thighs are parallel with the ground. Quickly return to the starting position, squeezing your glutes and thrusting your hips forward. Repeat at a quick pace. This exercise is going to tone your backside.

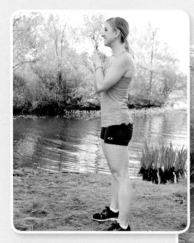

↑ **1.** Start standing tall with your feet shoulder-width apart and hands clasped in front of your chest.

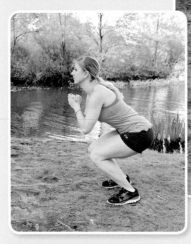

↑ **BAD:** Don't collapse your chest or let your knees bend in towards each other over your toes.

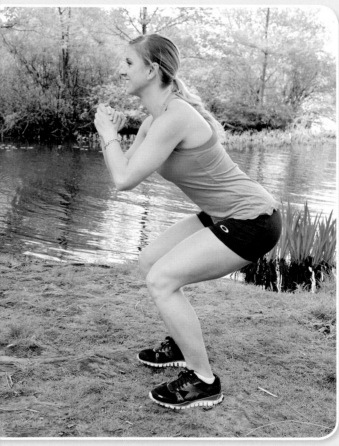

↑ **2.** Sit back onto your heels until your thighs are parallel with the ground.

CARDIO OPTION 2: 30-MINUTE PLYO-BARRE CARDIO ROUTINE

This workout is best to do between days of strength training. You do not need any equipment, and it requires little space, which makes it ideal for those who live in tiny apartments. You can, of course, do this outside as well. If you hate traditional cardiovascular exercise like running, this is also a good option for you, as it involves plyometric movements that raise the heart rate but are often followed by less intense moves to let you slightly recover. It includes a few of my favorite exercises from barre, boot-camp and kickboxing classes for a total-body burn that will leave you dripping with sweat.

MOVE 1:	Jog in Place
MOVE 2:	Speed Skaters
MOVE 3:	Jump Rope with Oblique Twists
MOVE 4:	Side-to-Side Ninja Kicks
MOVE 5:	In-and-Out Static Squat Jumps
MOVE 6:	Single-Leg Standing Crunches
MOVE 7:	Oblique Reach and Pull
MOVE 8:	Double Squat Jumps
MOVE 9:	Forward Jumping Jacks
MOVE 10:	Core Twist Jabs

Warm-up: Do each move for 30 seconds. This will allow your body to learn the movements and get comfortable while warming up the muscles.

Workout: Do each move for 1 minute without resting between moves. After you finish the tenth move, start back at the top and perform a second set for a total of 20 intense minutes of exercise. Perform each move as fast and explosively as you can. If you're jumping, see how high and far you can get.

Cooldown: Do each move again for 30 seconds to cool the body down. Take an extra second at the top or bottom of each move to feel your muscles elongate.

MOVE 1: **JOG IN PLACE**

Pump your arms as you bring your knees up toward your chest, mimicking a fast-paced jog on pavement or treadmill. The higher you get your knees, the more challenging it will be. You may also kick your butt with the heel of your foot for a little quad stretch as well. Start to warm up the body and raise your heart rate.

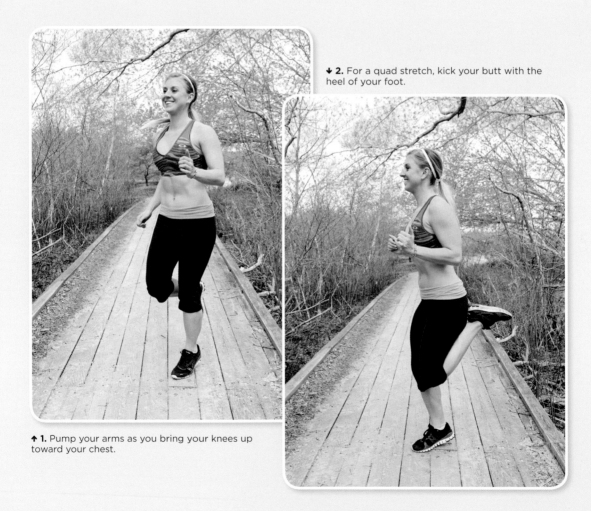

↓ **2.** For a quad stretch, kick your butt with the heel of your foot.

↑ **1.** Pump your arms as you bring your knees up toward your chest.

MOVE 2: **SPEED SKATERS**

Balance on a slightly bent right leg with left knee lifted in front of your body, your arms bent with your elbows by your sides, and your fists in front of your chest. Squat into your right heel and press through your glute to jump as far to the left as possible. Land gently on your left foot as you immediately lower yourself into a half squat and find your balance. Your right foot comes slightly behind your body, as if you were ice skating. Press through your left heel as you swing your right leg over, jumping as far as you can to the right. Repeat, jumping from side to side. Remember to keep your chest open and your eyes forward. Do not let your knee go beyond your toe when you sink down onto the balancing leg.

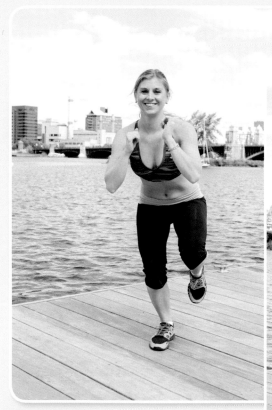

↑ **1.** Start by balancing on your right leg, knee slightly bent.

↓ **2.** Push off your right leg and hop as far as you can to your left, landing on a slightly bent left leg.

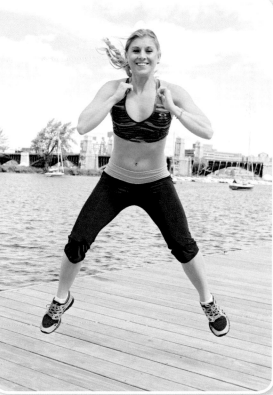

CARDIO OPTION 2

MOVE 3: **JUMP ROPE WITH OBLIQUE TWISTS**

Pretend to hold a jump rope in both hands. Quickly mimic the motions of jumping rope while rotating at the waist each time you lift off the ground. Your feet should be together, toes pointing in the same direction, alternating between 10 o'clock and 2 o'clock positions, as if your head were facing 12 o'clock. This move is great for getting a flatter tummy and reducing love handles.

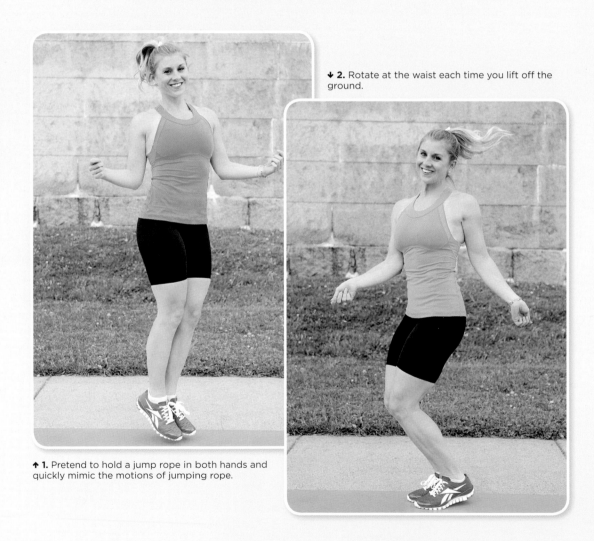

↓ **2.** Rotate at the waist each time you lift off the ground.

↑ **1.** Pretend to hold a jump rope in both hands and quickly mimic the motions of jumping rope.

54   SARAH FIT GET SKINNY AGAIN

MOVE 4: SIDE-TO-SIDE NINJA KICKS

Start with your hands in a ready position, arms bent at the elbow and your fists at chin level. As you bend your torso at the hips toward the right, kick your left foot out to the left with your foot flexed. Kick with your heel and get your foot as high as you can. As you lower your leg to the ground, stand up straight. Alternate now by bending at the hips to the left while kicking your right foot out to the side at hip height or higher. Continue alternating. Keep your torso straight and your arms in front of your chest the entire time. Do not bend at the waist. This is a total-body exercise that you'll feel in your lower body as well as your obliques.

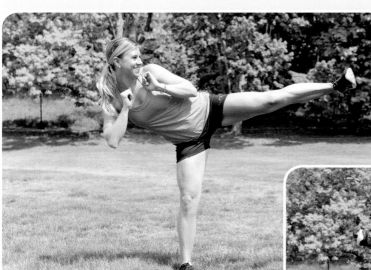

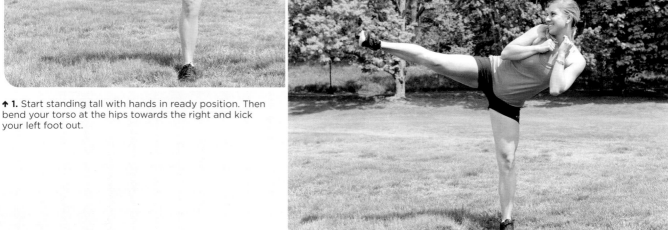

⬆ **1.** Start standing tall with hands in ready position. Then bend your torso at the hips towards the right and kick your left foot out.

⬇ **2.** Alternate by returning your left foot to the ground and then bending at the hips to the left while kicking your right foot out.

MOVE 5: **IN-AND-OUT STATIC SQUAT JUMPS**

Lower yourself into a squat position, fists in front of you and feet close together. Jump so that your feet are out wide into a sumo squat stance without changing the height of your head and torso. Immediately jump back to the starting position, feet together, again without changing the height of your head and torso. Jump quickly, your feet going in and out while maintaining the lower squat position. Do not let your back round down; keep your gaze looking forward and your chest open. The faster you go and the lower you squat, the more challenging this move will be. Your legs will be burning by the end of the interval, but don't stop!

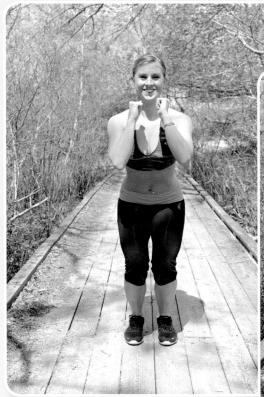

↑ 1. Lower yourself into a squat position.

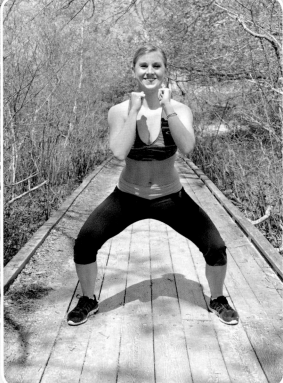

↓ 2. Jump so that your feet are wide in a sumo squat stance without changing the height of your head and torso.

MOVE 6: SINGLE-LEG STANDING CRUNCHES

Stand tall, with your back slightly arching backward, your right arm extended toward the sky, your left hand on your hip, a wall or a nearby railing. Extend your right leg, toes pointed, behind your body. Sweep your right knee in toward your chest at the same time you pull your right elbow down so that they contact each other. Extend your right arm back up and your right leg back behind your body quickly and rapidly repeat for 30 seconds before switching to the left side. For the 30-second intervals during the warm-up and cooldown, do each side for 15 seconds. As you bring your elbow down toward your navel, crunch your abs and pull your navel in toward your lower back. Breathe out each time your knee and elbow meet. This is another fabulous standing abs exercise that raises your heart rate.

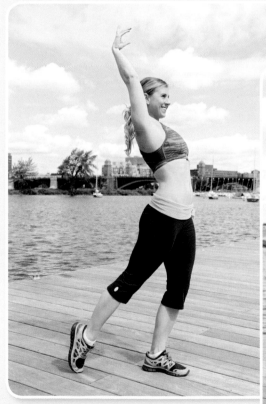

↑ **1.** Stand tall with your back slightly arching backward, your right arm extended toward the sky, left hand on your hip and your right leg pointed behind your body.

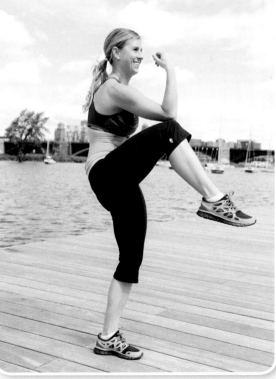

↓ **2.** Sweep your right knee in toward your chest at the same time you pull your right elbow down so they contact each other.

MOVE 7: **OBLIQUE REACH AND PULLS**

Start with your left hand on your hip, your right arm overhead, your right toes pointed and out to the side a few inches. Bring your right knee to meet your right elbow at the side while crunching your right obliques. Return your right foot back to start position and repeat quickly for 30 seconds before switching to the left side. For the 30-second intervals during warm-up and cooldown, do each side for 15 seconds. You're working your obliques here.

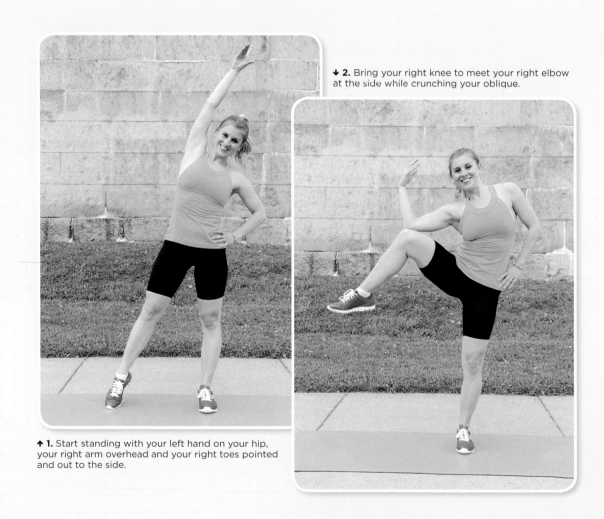

↓ 2. Bring your right knee to meet your right elbow at the side while crunching your oblique.

↑ 1. Start standing with your left hand on your hip, your right arm overhead and your right toes pointed and out to the side.

MOVE 8: **DOUBLE-SQUAT JUMPS**

With your feet hip width apart, lower yourself into a squat. Jump up as high as you can and softly land with your feet wide apart as you reach your left hand toward the ground, twisting to the right at the waist. Extend your right arm to the sky. Continue until your left hand touches the ground. Jump to bring your feet together as you lift your torso back to the starting position. Jump high and land with your feet wide apart as you touch the ground with your right arm, opening your chest up to the left while your left arm extends to the sky. Jump back to the starting position and quickly repeat. Keep your back flat during this exercise.

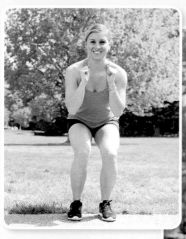

↑ **1.** Start with your feet hip width apart and lower yourself into a squat.

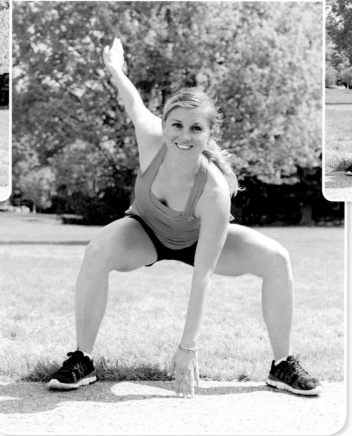

↑ **2.** Jump and land softly with your feet wide apart as you twist to the right at the waist and reach your left hand toward the ground.

↑ **3.** Jump back to starting position and repeat on the opposite side.

MOVE 9: FORWARD JUMPING JACKS

Start with your feet together, your arms out straight in front of your chest and your palms touching one another. Jump and land with your feet apart and open your arms to the sides at shoulder height, parallel with the ground. Hop, bringing your feet back together, as your hands clap in front of your chest. Jump in and out quickly, as you would if you were doing regular jumping jacks, as your arms open to the sides and close in front of your body.

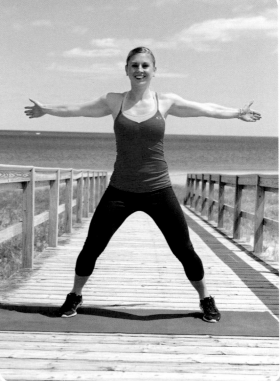

↓ **2.** Jump and land with your feet apart and your arms open to the sides.

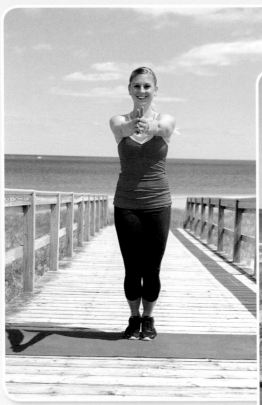

↑ **1.** Start with your feet together and your arms straight out in front of your chest with palms touching.

MOVE 10: CORE TWIST JABS

Start with knees bent, navel pulled in tight, spine straight. Bring both hands up in front of your face, fists at eye level. Quickly alternate punching with each hand. As you punch with the left, twist at your waist toward the right. As you punch with the right, twist your waist toward the left. Breathe out rapidly each time you punch forward. Keep knees gently bent the entire time and your core engaged. This is one of my favorite core exercises for creating definition and getting a flat stomach.

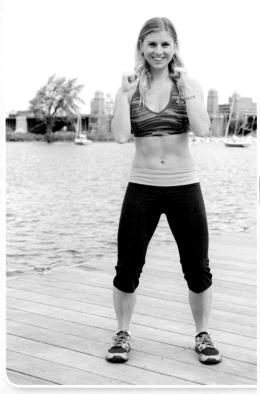

↑ 1. Start with knees bent and both hands up in front of your face, fists at eye level.

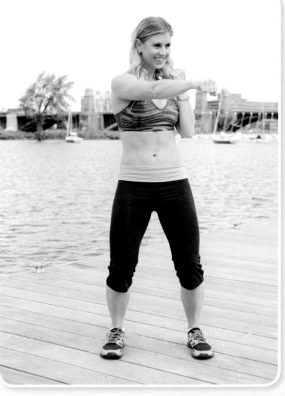

↓ 2. As you punch with your left hand, twist at your waist toward the right. Alternate between right and left jabs.

OUTDOOR RUNNING ROUTINES

Running is one of my favorite exercises. It is also one of the quickest ways to burn a ton of calories! You do not need any equipment, just a decent pair of running shoes. It can be done with a partner or group, fast or slow, long or short. When I run outdoors, my workouts go by faster and I'm able to train at a higher intensity. Remember to dress for your climate. Running in below-freezing temperatures is something many people actually enjoy! You just have to dress warm enough.

Intervals not only burn more fat and calories, but they also help improve your speed if you are planning to run a 5K or 10K in the near future. For some of the workouts, you will see a number from 5 to 10 that is called the RPE, or Rate of Perceived Exertion. The RPE is based on your personal effort or level of discomfort during an exercise or interval. You need to listen to your body when determining which level your are working at. A 10 is an all-out, intense effort and should be very hard. You shouldn't be able to maintain a 10 longer than 20 to 30 seconds. A 5 is an easy to moderate effort and should feel relatively easy. You should be able to maintain it for long period; this will also be your cooldown pace. As you lose weight and get in better shape, your levels will change. Your level 5 may go from a walk to a slow jog.

CARDIO OPTION 3: GET QUICK AND BURN FAT!

Warm up for 5 minutes at a slow to moderate pace. You are going to do 5 rounds of a 10–20–30-second interval. You will sprint for 10 seconds, run fast for 20 seconds and jog slowly for 30 seconds. You'll repeat this 10–20–30 interval 5 times for a total of 5 minutes. Afterward, you get to recover for 2 minutes with a walk or slow jog. If you are a beginner, learn to use your walk to catch your breath. After the 2 minutes are up, repeat the 10–20–30 series again for 5 rounds, followed by another 2-minute rest. Depending on your level of fitness, do 3 to 5 rounds total. Finish with a 5-minute cooldown. I do this workout using an interval timer on my smart phone. I currently use RunKeeper and have a video on YouTube that shows you how to do this.

5 minutes	Warm Up
10 seconds	Fast (9): almost all-out effort
20 seconds	Steady pace (8): keep intensity
30 seconds	Slow (6): recover at a slower jog
Do 4 more rounds for a total of 5, then recover for 2 minutes. Repeat the 7-minute sequence 4 more times, then cool down for 5 minutes at a slow jog.	

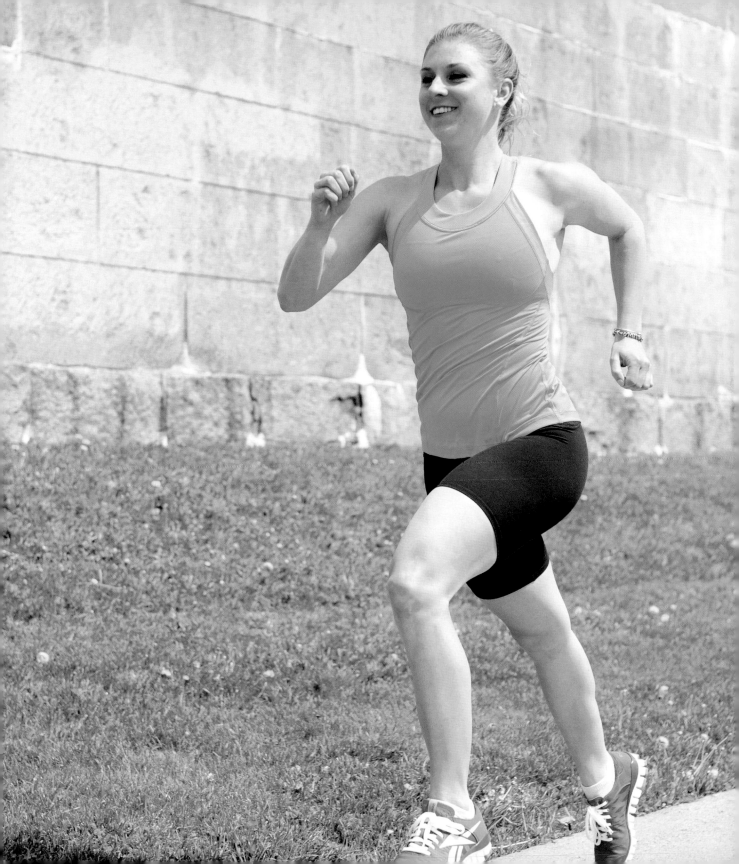

CARDIO OPTION 4: INTERVAL SONGS

If you do not have a smart phone or interval timer, the simplest way to do intervals is to use your playlist. Vary your intensity every other song, or on the basis of the beat of the song playing. Here is an example using some of my favorite all-time hits. Feel free to use your own pump-up beats.

Warm-up (5)	4:51	"I Wanna Dance with Somebody," by Whitney Houston
Fast (7)	3:32	"Pump It," by the Black Eyed Peas
Slower (6)	2:49	"Call on Me," by Eric Prydz
Fast (8)	3:56	"Rockafeller Skank," by Fatboy Slim
Slower (6)	4:25	"Dog Days Are Over," by Florence and the Machine
Fast (8)	4:18	"Maneater," by Nelly Furtado
Slower (6)	4:06	"I Made It," by Kevin Rudolf
Fast (9)	3:54	"Jetsetter," by Morningwood
Cooldown (5)	3:58	"Bleeding Love," by Leona Lewis

CARDIO OPTION 5: MINUTE TO WIN IT

The last outdoor running interval workout is for those who want to melt extra fat and have some running experience. This workout is not for the faint of heart. If you can push yourself to finish strong, not only will it burn a lot of calories but it will also help make you faster!

You're going to start out by running easily for 5 minutes to warm up. Next, you'll challenge yourself for 1 minute by running at a pace that you can barely maintain. Walk or jog slowly for 30 seconds to recover at a level 6. Repeat 2 more times. Fully recover for 5 minutes with a slow jog. If you are beginner, you may need to walk. Repeat the entire workout except for the warm-up 2 more times.

5 minutes	Warm-up	Easy (5)
BEGIN INTERVAL WORKOUT		
1 minute	Run fast	Hard (7)
30 seconds	Walk	Moderate (6)
1 minute	Run fast	Hard (8)
30 seconds	Walk	Moderate (6)
1 minute	Run fast	Hard (9)
30 seconds	Walk	Moderate (6)
5 minutes	Slow jog	Moderate (5–6)

Repeat the interval workout 2 more times all the way through. During the 30-second walks, really try to catch your breath. You should not feel fully recovered by the end of the 30 seconds. If you do, you are not running fast enough during the minute sprint. You probably will not be able to maintain a sprint for the full 60 seconds, but that doesn't mean you should not try. You get to walk afterward! By the end of the 5-minute slow jog, you should feel close to fully recovered and ready for another round.

STRETCHING

It's important to stretch for about 5 minutes after a challenging strength workout to prevent muscle soreness, but it's also a good idea to fit in a longer stretch session as least once a week. This may be a yoga class you do at your leisure or a series of moves done next to your bed as soon as you get up in the morning or on the floor while watching TV. My at home stretching sequence is inspired by my favorite yoga poses. Do them in silence or put on your favorite Rihanna jam. I love to do this routine on mornings when I have to wake up early. It helps build energy for the day.

If you prefer classes or following along to videos, I have a variety of stretching sequences on my YouTube channel. For your stretch day, do this sequence or the stretching series in the gym section, take a yoga class or pick one of my YouTube videos. You can go through the moves quickly for a post-workout stretch, but I encourage you to take some time, pausing for at least 5 full breaths in each position.

YOGA STRETCH AT HOME

Begin the sequence marching in place. Moves 2–17 are done on one side of the body. When you reach move 17, return to move 2 and go through sequence on the opposite side of the body. Finish with moves 18–21.

YOGA STRETCH AT HOME

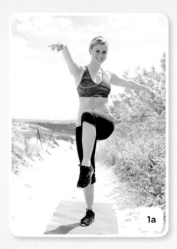
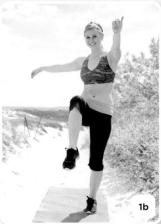

Move 1. March in Place with Swinging Arms: swing your arms freely as you march in place, bringing your knees as high as you can. Keep your stomach engaged.

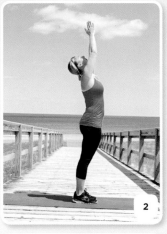

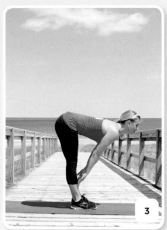

Move 2. Mountain Pose: stand up tall with your palms pressed together, arms up over your head and reaching behind you with your back slightly arched.

Move 3. Fold Over: bring your hands down to the ground with a flat back and touch your hands to the floor.

Move 4. High Plank: plant your hands on the ground and step your feet back into a high-plank position.

Move 5. Cobra: lower your chest and the rest of your body slowly to the ground from the high-plank position and then gently press your chest up off the ground and reach it forward.

Move 6. Downward Dog: tuck your toes under and raise your hips up off the ground and press into your heels with your head between your biceps. Press your chest away from your hands with your fingers spread. Press your shoulder blades down, away from your ears, and keep your back straight.

Move 7. Downward Dog Split: lift your right leg up toward the sky, keeping hips level.

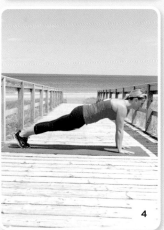

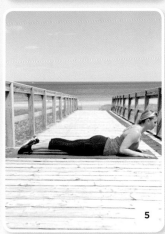

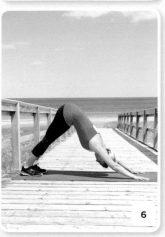

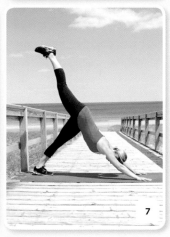

YOGA STRETCH AT HOME

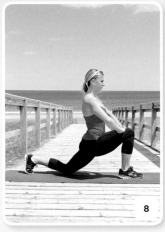

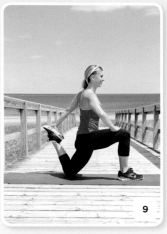

Move 8. Low Lunge: bring your right leg in toward your chest and plant your foot between your hands. Rise up into a high lunge.

Move 9. Quad Stretch: lift your left foot toward your glutes and grab your ankle if you can with your left hand, stretching your left quadriceps.

Move 10. Hip Flexor Stretch: let go of your ankle and form a 90-degree angle with your right knee. Press your left hip forward, your left arm reaching up and over slightly to the right.

Move 11. Hamstring Stretch: with your left leg in a 90-degree angle, extend your right leg out straight and bend over reaching for your toes and feeling a stretch in the hamstring.

Move 12. Cat Cow: come into a tabletop position on all fours, your hands directly below your shoulders and knees directly under hips. Take a deep breath in and tilt your head back and look up as you lift your tailbone up toward the sky. Your back will be concave. As you exhale, tilt your tailbone down toward the ground and round your back, spreading your shoulders blades apart. Feel a stretch across your back and allow your head to hang down toward the ground. Inhale and exhale for 5 full breaths.

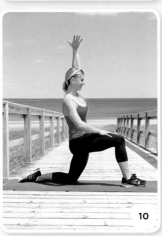

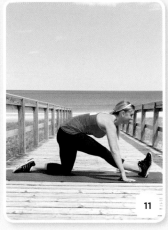

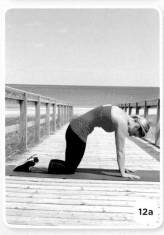

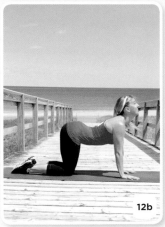

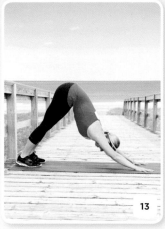

13

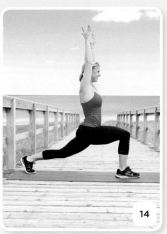

14

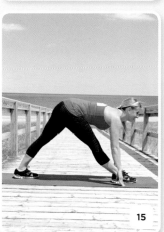

15

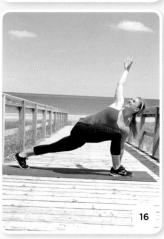

16

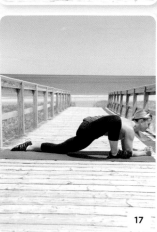

17

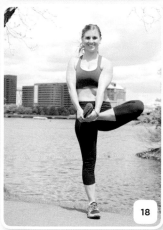

18

Move 13. Downward Dog: curl your toes under and press your back into a downward dog. Repeat the sequence, starting from the low lunge on the opposite side.

Move 14. High Lunge: from the downward dog, bring your right foot to between your hands on the floor. Raise your arms up into a high lunge with your fingertips pointing toward the sky, your front knee bent and your knee in line with your ankle, your back knee up off the ground.

Move 15. Forward Fold-Over Triangle: straighten your front leg and bend at the hips, folding your torso over your front leg while fully stretching your right leg behind you. This should feel amazing if you have tight hamstrings.

Move 16. Torso-Twist Lunge: rebend your front knee and place your left hand beside your right foot. Open your chest up toward the right, reaching your right arm up toward the sky. Feel a stretch all across the front of your chest. Keep your navel pulled in tight toward your spine. Keep your back knee up off the ground.

Move 17. Low-Lunge Hip Opener: place your left knee back down on the ground. Position both forearms on the ground to the left of your right foot. Let your right knee fall to the left side, lifting up the sole of your right foot so that you are balancing on the outer edge of your right foot, forearms and left knee. Feel a stretch in your right hip and just rest. Repeat this sequence, starting in the high-lunge position on the opposite side.

Move 18. Standing-Side Butt Stretch: standing up tall, balence on your left heel and bring your right ankle across your left knee. Hold your right foot slightly higher than knee height on your left leg. Keep your chest open and your back straight. You should feel a stretch in the outside of your right glute. Gently press your right knee down toward the ground for a deeper stretch. Repeat on the opposite side.

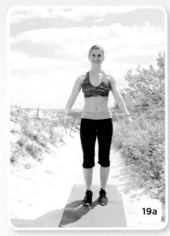
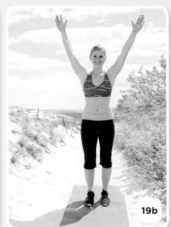

19a

19b

Move 19. Arm Circles: stand up tall with your arms by your sides, pressing your shoulders away from ears. Sweep your arms up overhead in a circular motion. Pretend to draw a large circle with your fingertips, keeping your shoulders pressed down and away from your ears the entire time.

Move 20. Triceps Stretch: standing up tall, place your right hand behind your head with your bicep close to your ear. Take your left hand and gently press down on your right elbow as you bring it closer to the center of your head. You should feel a stretch along your right triceps muscle. To make this move more advanced, take your left hand and reach for your right hand behind your back. You may do this move holding onto a towel as well if you can't quite reach your hands together.

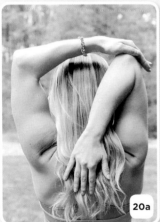
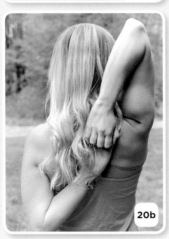

20a

20b

Move 21. Chest Opener: stand up tall with your knees slightly bent and your hands clasped behind your back, arms straight. Bend at the hips and let your chest fall onto your thighs if it reaches. Let your arms hang over behind your head for a chest stretch. Then bend your right knee and bring your right shoulder to meet it as your chest opens up to the left looking out over your left shoulder. Pause for 1–2 breaths and switch to the opposite side.

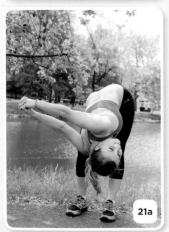
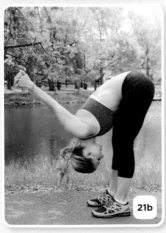

21a

21b

LONG DAY

One day a week, I want you to push yourself to exercise longer than you are comfortable with. If you are training for a race like a half marathon, this is ideal, but if you are just trying to lose weight, it's great for burning off extra stored energy, especially if you had a big night out or binge during the week.

How long should you work out, and what should you do? If you love to run, go for a long, easy run. It doesn't have to be super-intense, but go for more than what you usually do. For example, if you usually run for 40 minutes, try 60 minutes.

If this sounds like a lot, don't worry, there are plenty of options below depending on your fitness level.

Option 1: Take an easy, long run or bike ride for 60–90 minutes. If you're running, feel free to take breaks, walking as often as you need.

Option 2: Alternate between running and walking at 5-minute intervals for 60 minutes.

Option 3: Do two of the indoor cardio workouts (pages 98-101) with a 5-minute break between sets.

Option 4: Plan a ski trip or a hike, go kayaking, explore a new city on foot while sightseeing, rent a stand-up paddleboard for an hour or engage is some other activity with a group of friends. You'll be having fun and won't realize all the calories you are burning.

If you don't love what you are doing, you are not going to be inspired to make it a habit. Make fitness a part of your life. Option 4 is my favorite, so I encourage you to try to plan as many activities as possible throughout the year.

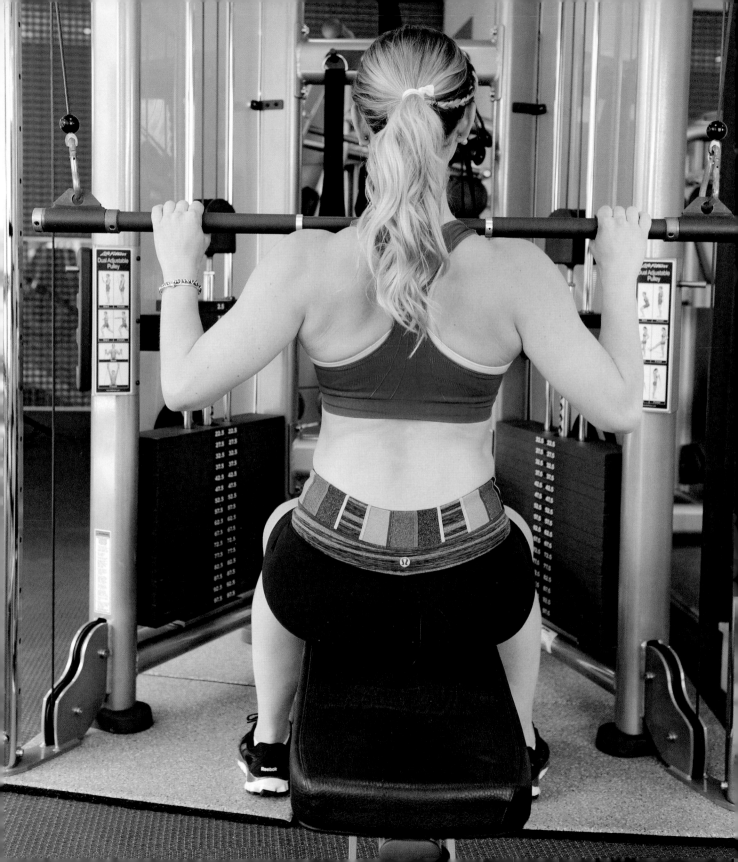

CHAPTER 2

TIME TO HIT THE GYM

Though you can certainly lose weight and tone up without it, the gym is where you will be able to make some of the most fitness gains. Adding resistance, instability and variety will keep your body from getting comfortable and allow you to continue to transform it. There are thousands of exercises you can do, but I've chosen my favorite moves that have proven successful in my own training.

I've left out the tricky ones that can cause injury if performed incorrectly. If you have a favorite move, go ahead and add it, or modify my moves when appropriate. When performing any strength exercise, deliberately squeeze the muscle that you are working at the peak range of motion. This extra bit of work will help you see results faster and ensure that the correct muscle is being used for the exercise.

If you love to take group exercise classes at your gym or in a studio, go ahead and take classes that correspond with your fitness plan. For example, take a spin class on a cardiovascular day or try a barre class on a strength day. Variation in your plan will prevent you from getting bored and keep you on track to getting skinny again.

SCHEDULE

DAY 1:	Strength	DAY 5:	Strength or yoga/stretch
DAY 2:	Cardiovascular	DAY 6:	Long day
DAY 3:	Strength	DAY 7:	Off
DAY 4:	Cardiovascular		

STRENGTH TRAINING

Strength training at the gym is one of the fastest ways to tone up your body. The ability to really fatigue your muscles quickly will yield the fastest results. The leanest I have ever been came from heavy lifting 2 or 3 times a week, and minimal running. I was shocked, but the science doesn't lie. Heavy lifting will not make you bulky. It will build muscle, burn fat and leave you looking sexy and fabulous.

Below is one of my favorite workouts, and it will leave you sore!

TOTAL BODY BLAST: STRENGTH TRAINING AT THE GYM 1

You may need to do this workout a couple of times to find the right weight for each exercise. I encourage you *not* to use the same set of dumbbells for each exercise, as your strength varies from one muscle group to another. Your legs are much stronger than your arms. If you are doing bicep curls with 8-pound/4-kg dumbbells, you should be doing deadlifts with at least 12.5-pound/6-kg weights. The weights given are just a suggestion. Please adjust for your own level of strength.

Do each exercise for the number of reps recommended. Your muscles should be fatigued by the last rep. Move on to the next exercise without resting . If you need a sip of water, go for it; otherwise, grab the equipment that you need and get moving! The less rest, the more calories you'll burn. Do the first circuit 3 times through, resting for one minute between sets. The first circuit focuses on the upper body. The second circuit is dedicated to the lower body. The last circuit is geared toward firming up your midsection.

CIRCUIT 1:

You will need a medium and heavy set of dumbbells as well as a physioball.

MOVE 1:	Bicep Curl Balances (5–12 lb/2–6 kg dumbbells), 15–20 reps
MOVE 2:	Triceps Dip with Physioball, 12–15 reps
MOVE 3:	Chest Presses on Physioball (10–15 lb/5–7 kg dumbbells), 15–20 reps
MOVE 4:	Bent-Over Rows (10-15 lb/5–7 kg dumbbells), 12–15 reps
Rest for 1 minute and repeat this circuit 2 more times, including the rest.	

CIRCUIT 2:

You will need a heavy and medium set of dumbbells, Bosu ball and step or bench.

MOVE 5:	Bosu Ball Push-Ups with Overhead Press, 12–15 reps
MOVE 6:	Dumbbell Swings (10-20 lb/5-10 kg dumbbell), 12–15 reps
MOVE 7:	Step-Ups (8-15 lb/4-7 kg dumbbells), 12–15 reps
MOVE 8:	Single-Leg Deadlifts (10-15 lb/5-7 kg dumbbells), 12–15 reps
Rest for 1 minute and repeat this circuit 2 more times, including the rest.	

CIRCUIT 3:

You will need a dumbbell and physioball.

MOVE 9:	Russian Twist with dumbbell (5-10 lb/2-5 kg dumbbell), 15 reps
MOVE 10:	Physioball Jackknifes, 8 reps
MOVE 11:	Physioball Side Crunches, 10 reps on each side
MOVE 12:	Dumbbell V-ups (5-10 lb/2-5 kg dumbbell), 8 reps
Rest for 1 minute and repeat this circuit 2 more times, including the rest.	

MOVE 1: **BICEP CURL BALANCES**

Stand tall, balanced on one foot and with 8–10 lb/4–5 kg dumbbells in your hands. Your arms should hang down in front of body, the backs of your hands grazing your thighs. Lift the dumbbells up toward your armpits and slowly lower them back down. Switch to balance on the other leg halfway through the set.

TIP: Raise the dumbbells for a count of 1 and lower them slowly for a count of 3 for extra burn. This exercise is going to give you some sexy guns to show off.

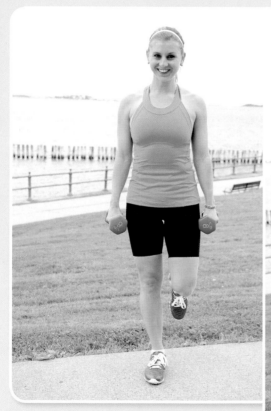

↑ **1.** Stand tall, balanced on one foot with dumbbells in your hands.

↓ **2.** Lift the dumbbells up toward your armpits and slowly lower them back down.

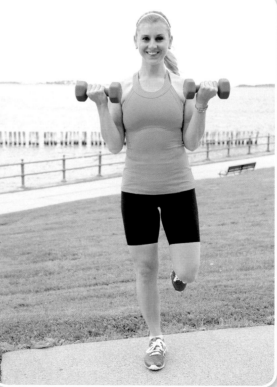

MOVE 2: **TRICEPS DIPS WITH PHYSIOBALL**

Start with your butt on a bench and the palms of your hands placed on its edge. Balance your feet on top of a physioball. Lift your butt off the bench and lower your hips toward the ground, keeping your feet balanced on the physioball. Press through the heels of your hands until your arms are completely straight. Repeat.

TIP: Keep your spine as close to the bench as possible. If this is too hard, place your feet on the floor and remove the physioball.

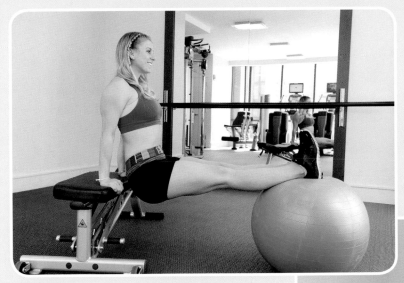

2. Lift your butt off the bench and lower your hips toward the ground, keeping your feet balanced on the physioball.

1. Start with your butt on a bench and the palms of your hands placed on its edge. Balance your feet on top of a physioball.

MOVE 3: CHEST PRESSES ON PHYSIOBALL

Place your upper back on a physioball, your butt, knees and chest in a straight line. Engage your core and squeeze your glutes while holding a 10-15 lb/5-7 kg dumbbell in each hand next to your shoulders. Press the dumbbells up to meet each other above your chin while your body remains still. Slowly lower the dumbbells back to the starting position. This move is great for keeping your chest looking perky.

TIP: If this move is too challenging, eliminate the physioball and do it on a workout bench.

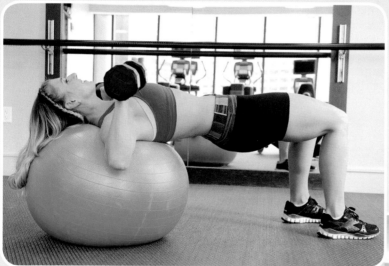

↑ **1.** Place your upper back on a physioball, your butt, knees and chest in a straight line while holding a dumbbell in each hand.

↓ **2.** Press the dumbbells up to meet each other above your chin while your body remains still.

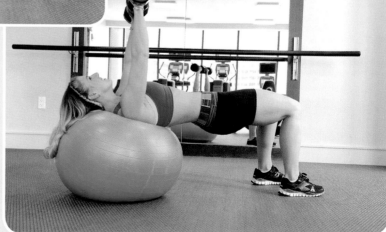

MOVE 4: **BENT-OVER ROWS**

Start with your feet hip width apart, slightly bent from the hips and your torso leaning forward at a 45-degree angle. Engage your core as if someone were about to punch you in the gut. Hold a 10-15 lb/5-7 kg dumbbell in each hand with your palms facing each other, your arms extended downward so that the weights are just above knee height. Squeeze your shoulder blades together and bring the weights up to your waist as you pull your shoulder blades down and away from your ears. Slowly lower the weights back to the starting position. This exercise strengthens your back and will help alleviate back pain as well as reduce back fat.

TIP: Make sure you squeeze your shoulder blades together, using the muscles in your back to lift the weights.

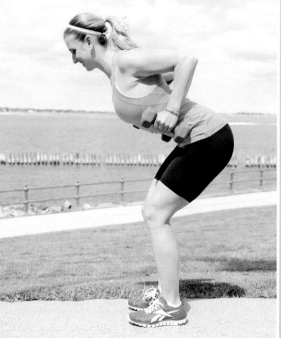

↓ **2.** Squeeze your shoulder blades together and bring the weights up to your waist.

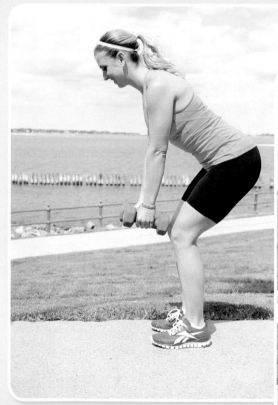

↑ **1.** With a dumbbell in each hand, start with your feet hip width apart, slightly bent from the hips and your torso leaning forward at a 45-degree angle.

MOVE 5: **BOSU BALL PUSH-UPS WITH OVERHEAD PRESS**

Start in a high-plank position with your hands on the outsides of a Bosu ball, the rounded surface facing the ground. Your body should form a straight line from shoulders to ankles. Lower your body into a push-up and press back up to plank position. Jump, bringing your feet in toward the Bosu ball. Stand up, lifting the Bosu ball overhead and keeping your arms straight the entire time. Slowly lower the Bosu back to the ground. This move works your core, shoulders, chest and lower body. It's a total-body fat burner by itself!

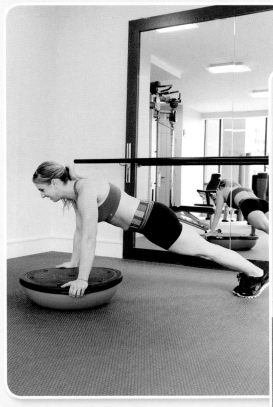

↑ 1. Start in a high-plank position with your hands on the outsides of a Bosu ball.

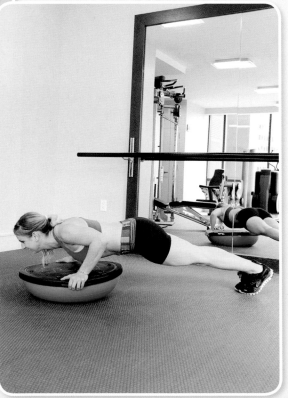

↓ 2. Lower your body into a push-up and press back up to plank position.

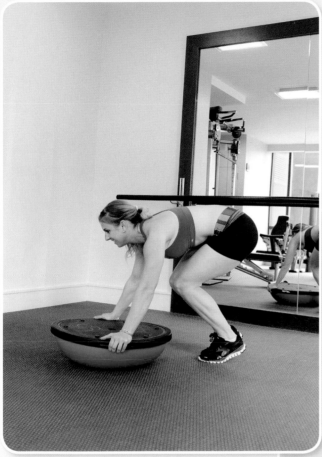

↑ 3. Jump, bringing your feet in toward the Bosu ball.

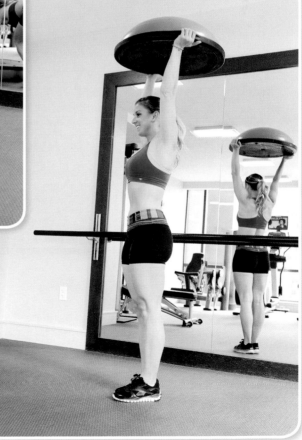

↓ 4. Stand up, lifting the Bosu ball overhead and keeping your arms straight the entire time.

MOVE 6: **DUMBBELL SWINGS**

Stand with your legs wider than hip width apart. Holding a 10–20 lb/5–9 kg kettlebell or a dumbbell with both hands, grab it in the middle and extend your arms down the front of your body. Press your hips back and bend your knees, bringing the kettlebell or dumbbell between and slightly behind your legs. Thrust your hips forward as you straighten up, bringing the dumbbell up to shoulder height using momentum, not your shoulder muscles.

TIP: Remember to keep your back straight. Do not round your shoulders. Also avoid excessively swinging the dumbbell. Keep it controlled and no higher than your shoulders.

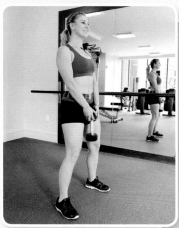

↑ **1.** Stand with your legs wider than hip width apart while holding a dumbbell with both hands down the front of your body.

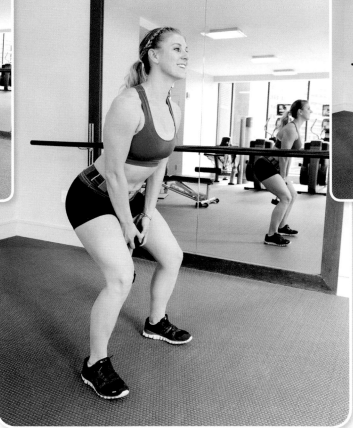

↑ **3.** Thrust your hips forward as you straighten up, bringing the dumbbell up to shoulder height.

↑ **2.** Press your hips back and bend your knees, bringing the dumbbell between and slightly behind your legs.

MOVE 7: **STEP-UPS**

Standing in front of a bench that is mid-shin to knee height with a pair of dumbbells weighing 8–15 lb/4–7 kg in your hands. Raise one foot onto the bench, pressing through your heel to bring the opposite foot up onto the bench as well. Lower one foot at a time, starting with the foot you stepped up with. Repeat all reps on the same side before switching.

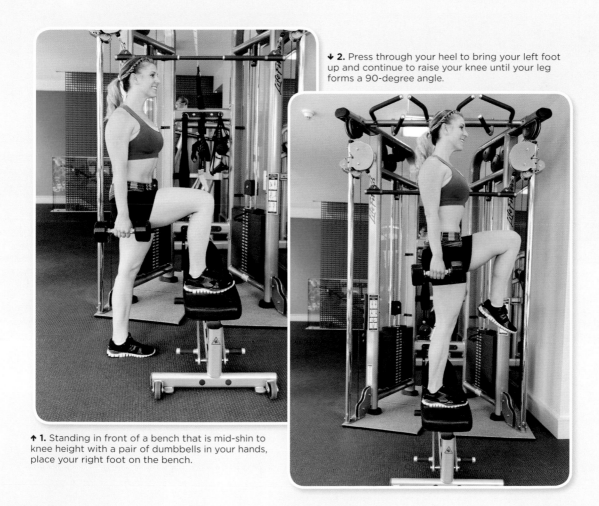

↓ **2.** Press through your heel to bring your left foot up and continue to raise your knee until your leg forms a 90-degree angle.

↑ **1.** Standing in front of a bench that is mid-shin to knee height with a pair of dumbbells in your hands, place your right foot on the bench.

MOVE 8: **SINGLE-LEG DEADLIFTS**

Standing tall with a pair of 10–15 lb/5–7 kg dumbbells in your hands, balance on your right leg, the left one straight with foot flexed, slightly lifted behind your body. Bend forward at the waist, keeping the dumbbells close to your legs and your back straight. As your torso falls forward, let your left leg ride up like a seesaw so that your body forms a straight line from your shoulders to your left ankle. Engage your right glute and return to the starting position. Do all reps on one side and then switch legs.

TIP: Make sure your back stays straight the entire time. As you lift your left leg, make sure to feel a stretch in the back of the right leg. Engage the bottom of your right glute to lift your torso back to starting position. This exercise hits your entire backside, including back, butt and hamstrings.

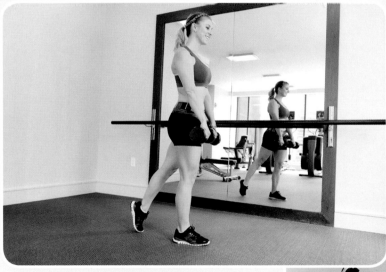

↑ **1.** Standing tall with a pair of dumbbells in your hands, balance on your right leg, the left one straight, slightly behind your body.

↓ **2.** Bend forward at the waist and let your left leg ride up like a seesaw so that your body forms a straight line.

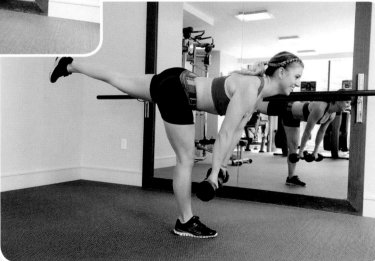

MOVE 9: **RUSSIAN TWISTS WITH DUMBBELL**

Sit on your tailbone with your knees bent and your feet slightly lifted off the ground. Your chest should be open and your torso straight and leaning slightly back. Hold a medicine ball or 4-10 lb/ 2-5 kg dumbbell with both hands in front of your navel. Rotate your shoulders to the right, twisting at your waist and bringing the dumbbell to the right. Exhale and bring the dumbbell to the opposite side, again twisting at the waist. This move helps get rid of those dreaded love handles.

TIP: Make this harder by letting your knees fall to the side opposite from the direction in which your torso is turning.

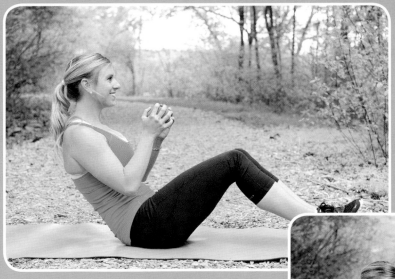

↑ **1.** Sit on your tailbone with your knees bent and your feet slightly lifted off the ground. Hold the dumbbell with both hands in front of your navel.

↓ **2.** Rotate your shoulders to the right, twisting at your waist and bring the dumbbell to the right.

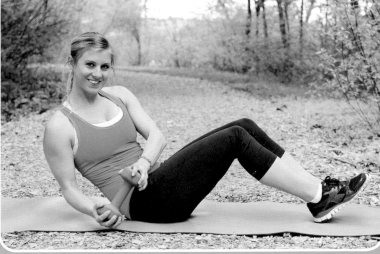

MOVE 10: **PHYSIOBALL JACKKNIFES**

Place the tops of your feet on a physioball and walk your hands out until you are balancing in a high-plank position with your feet on top of the ball. Exhale and bring your feet and the ball in toward your chest. Fully extend your legs to return to the starting position. This is one challenging core move. You can do it.

TIP: Do not let your hips rise up too high when you bring the ball into toward your chest. As you return to the starting position, don't let your hips sink down, either.

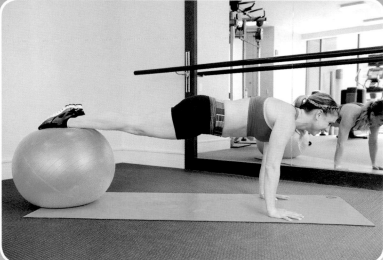

↑ **1.** Place the tops of your feet on a physioball and walk your hands out until you are balancing in a high-plank position.

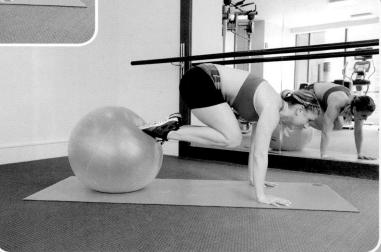

↓ **2.** Bring your feet and the ball in toward your chest. Fully extend your legs to return to the starting position.

MOVE 11: **PHYSIOBALL SIDE CRUNCHES**

Sit on a physioball, facing a wall. Turn your feet to the right, placing them against the floor where it meets the wall. Balance on your right hip. Bend at your hips and lower your torso toward the ground. You should not hit the ball as long as it is placed low enough on your hip, but high enough for you to balance. Raise your torso back to the starting position, crunching your left obliques and slightly rotating your left shoulder open. Do all reps on one side before switching sides.

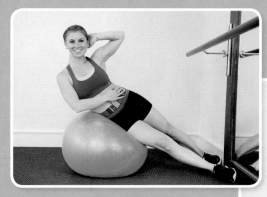

↑ 1. Sit on a physio ball, facing a wall. Turn your feet to the right, placing them against the floor where it meets the wall.

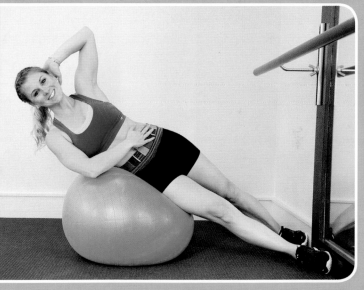

↑ 2. Bend at your hips and lower your torso toward the ground.

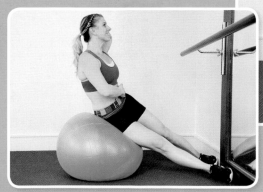

↑ 3. Raise your torso back up, crunching your left obliques and slightly rotating your left shoulder open.

MOVE 12: **DUMBBELL V-UPS**

Sit, balancing on your tailbone with legs in tabletop position while holding a 5-10 lb/2-5 kg dumbbell in front of your chest. Take a deep breath in and on the exhale, slowly lower your back toward the ground while straightening out your legs, making sure not to touch the ground. Hold for 1 count and return to starting position.

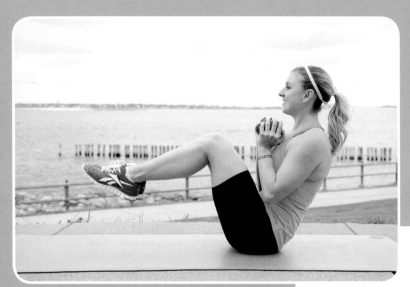

↓ 2. Slowly lower your back toward the ground while straightening out your legs, making sure not to touch the ground.

↑ 1. Sit, balancing on your tailbone with legs in tabletop position while holding a dumbbell in front of your chest.

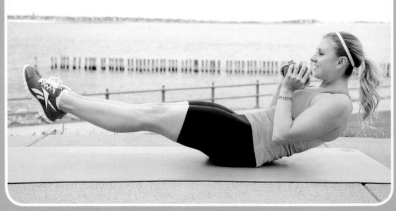

STRENGTH TRAINING AT THE GYM 2

Some of my biggest gains when it comes to muscle have come in the gym. Without the heavier weights, I never would have seen those gains. Every person is different and responds to a strength routine on the basis of genetic predisposition. I tend to gain muscle fairly easily. I will never look like a she-male, but I can gain a couple of pounds of muscle in a few months with proper training.

Some people will find it very difficult to put on the smallest amount of muscle to help create definition. If this is you, try this workout regularly and challenge yourself with the weights. You should barely be able to squeeze out the last repetition. If you are not struggling to finish, then increase the weight. I give weight suggestions, but do not be afraid to go heavier or lighter depending on your ability.

This routine replicates the routine that I did to lose 100% of my excess body fat. It was a time in my life when I was doing the least amount of cardio and the most strength training. Do not be afraid of the strength routines. They are going to give you the most visible results! Do these 6 moves back-to-back. Rest for 30 to 45 seconds between each move when you first start out. As you progress, reduce the rest time until you are no longer resting at all. To warm up, do a quick mini set consisting of 5 reps of each move to get familiar with the movement before adding weight. Remember to stretch after this workout.

MOVE 1:	Lateral Pull-Downs, 12–15 reps
MOVE 2:	Seated Low Rows, 12–15 reps
MOVE 3:	Walking Lunges with Bicep Curls (8-12 lb/3.6-5.4 kg dumbbells), 12-15 reps
MOVE 4:	Triceps Extensions (5-15 lb/2.3-6.8 kg dumbbells), 12–15 reps
MOVE 5:	Ball-Pass Crunches, 12–15 reps
MOVE 6:	Sumo-Squat Shoulder Presses (5-15 lb/2.3-6.8 kg dumbbells), 12–15 reps

Do each exercise back-to-back, resting 30–45 seconds between exercises. After you've done each exercise once, start back at the top and repeat 2 additional times for 3 sets total.

MOVE 1: **LATERAL PULL-DOWNS**

Suggested weight: 40–60 lbs/18–27.2 kg

Sit down on a workout bench with your hands slightly wider than shoulder width apart, grasping a cable bar that is just high enough that your arms are fully stretched. Pressing your shoulders away from your ears, use your back muscles to pull the bar down toward your chest. Keep your core engaged and squeeze your shoulder blades together. Your elbows should come down to your sides and the cable bar should be right underneath your chin. Slowly raise the bar back to the starting position.

TIP: This move will give you sexy back definition. Don't have a cable machine? Hold a dumbbell in each hand and bend forward at the hips. Let the dumbbells sit on top of your thighs. Bring the weights in toward your waist as you squeeze your shoulder blades together and away from your ears. Slowly return to the starting position. Pull from your back, not your arms.

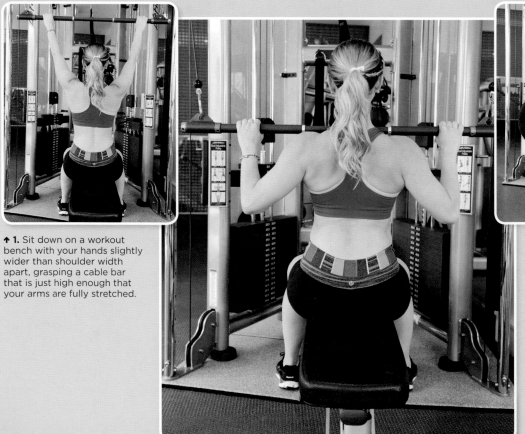

↑ **1.** Sit down on a workout bench with your hands slightly wider than shoulder width apart, grasping a cable bar that is just high enough that your arms are fully stretched.

↑ **3.** If you don't have a cable machine, try the bent-over dumbbell row instead.

← **2.** Pressing your shoulders away from your ears, use your back muscles to pull the bar down toward your chest.

MOVE 2: **SEATED LOW ROWS**

Suggested weight: 30–40 lbs/13.6–18 kg

Sit on a bench facing a cable machine. Position the pulley slightly lower than your seated chest height. Stretch your arms forward to grab hold of the close grip handle. Sit with your back straight and core engaged. Press your shoulders down, away from your ears. Pull the handle toward your navel using your back muscles and squeezing your shoulder blades together. Try to pull your shoulders back as well by really squeezing all your back muscles. Slowly return to the starting position.

TIP: Don't have a cable machine? Try doing this move with a resistance band around the balls of your feet while sitting up tall and holding onto the ends. This move is going to improve your posture and help you stand up taller.

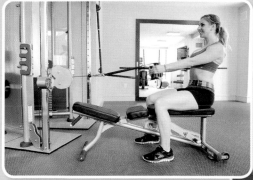

↑ **1.** Sit on a bench facing a cable machine and stretch your arms forward to grab hold of the grip handle.

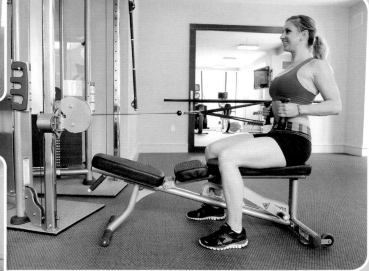

↑ **2.** Pull the handle toward your navel using your back muscles and squeezing your shoulder blades together.

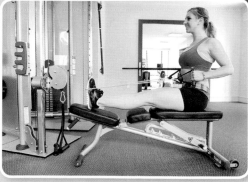

↑ **3.** If you don't have a cable machine, try doing this move with a resistance band around the balls of your feet.

MOVE 3: WALKING LUNGES WITH BICEP CURLS

Suggested weight: 8–12 lbs/3.6–5.4 kg

Start by standing up tall. Take a big step forward and lower yourself into a lunge with the weights down by your sides. As you press through from your heel to stand back up, bring the dumbbells up toward your armpits with your palms facing your chest. Balance on one leg before stepping forward with the foot still lifted and then stepping right into another lunge.

TIP: If your lower body is stronger than your upper, you may do a bicep curl every other lunge.

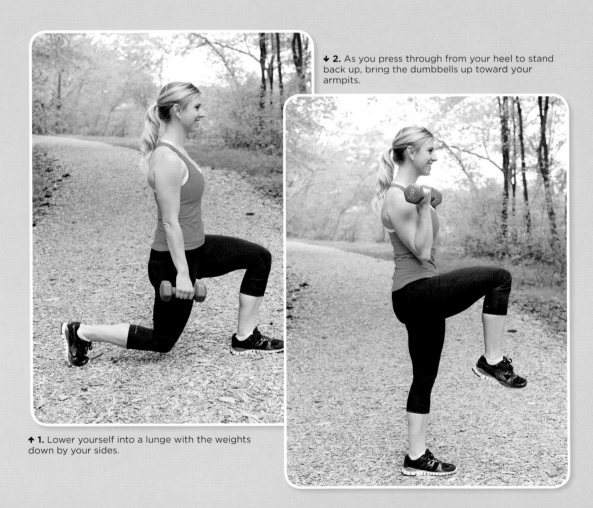

↓ **2.** As you press through from your heel to stand back up, bring the dumbbells up toward your armpits.

↑ **1.** Lower yourself into a lunge with the weights down by your sides.

MOVE 4: **TRICEPS EXTENSIONS**

Suggested weight: 5–15 lbs/2.3–6.8 kg

Sit cross-legged on the floor with a single dumbbell held by both hands directly behind your head. Keep your biceps close to your ears and your back straight. Extend your arms up toward the sky, bringing the weight overhead using your triceps. Slowly lower the weight back down.

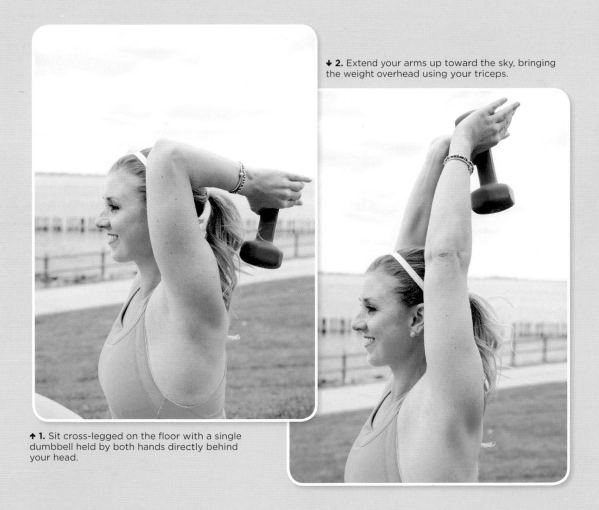

↓ 2. Extend your arms up toward the sky, bringing the weight overhead using your triceps.

↑ 1. Sit cross-legged on the floor with a single dumbbell held by both hands directly behind your head.

MOVE 5: **BALL-PASS CRUNCHES**

Lying on your back on the ground, place a physioball between your hands and fully extend your legs about 6 inches/15 cm off of the ground. Lift your shoulder blades up off the ground to reach for your feet with the ball. Place the ball between your feet and start to lower both legs toward the ground as you lower your shoulder blades back to the ground. Continue to lower your legs until your abs start to pop up off the ground, about 6–12 inches/15–30 cm above the floor. Try to keep your abs pressed into the ground. Breathe out and bring your legs back to starting position as you lift your shoulder blades off of the ground to grab the ball. Continue passing the ball between feet and hands.

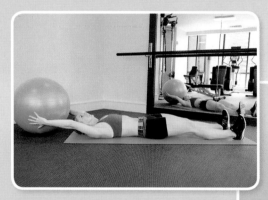

↑ 1. Lie on your back on the ground with a physioball between your hands.

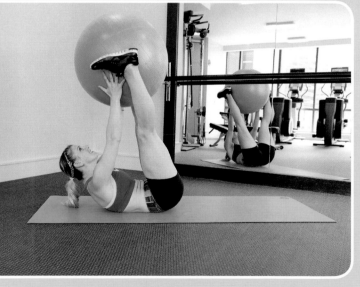

↑ 2. Fully extend your legs off of the ground and lift your shoulder blades up off the ground to reach for your feet with the ball.

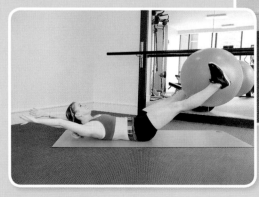

↑ 3. Place the ball between your feet and start to lower both legs toward the ground as you lower your shoulder blades back to the ground.

MOVE 6: **SUMO-SQUAT SHOULDER PRESSES**

Suggested weight: 5–15 lbs/2.3–6.8 kg

Stand tall with, feet wider than shoulder width apart, toes pointed toward 2 o'clock and 10 o'clock. Hold a pair of dumbbells close to your chest with your palms facing each other at shoulder height. Lower yourself into a squat until your thighs are parallel with the ground. Your knees should be in line with your ankles. As you rise back up, press the weights up overhead, keeping your ears between your biceps and your palms facing one another. Slowly lower your arms to starting position.

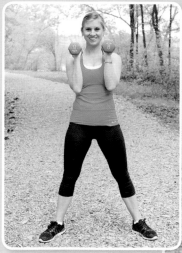

↑ **1.** Standing tall with feet wider than shoulder width apart, hold a pair of dumbbells close to your chest at shoulder height.

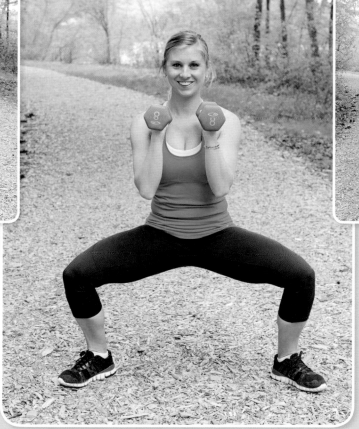

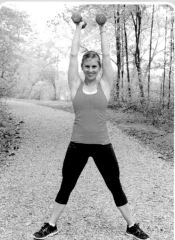

↑ **3.** As you rise back up, press the weights up overhead.

↑ **2.** Lower yourself into a squat until your thighs are parallel with the ground.

CARDIO

Access to a gym will keep your cardio routine extra spicy. In addition to the workouts I give you in this chapter, I encourage you to try a group exercise class like spinning, kickboxing, Zumba or another dance class on days that are designated for cardio.

Never stepped into a gym before? You will find a variety of machines, such as treadmills, stair-climbers, elliptical machines, arch trainers, spin bikes, seated bikes and more. Here is a quick breakdown of my favorites.

Elliptical: This machine is one of the most popular for good reason. It gives you an upper-body and lower-body workout at the same time. If you have bad knees, it's also easy on your joints because it is a low-impact machine. The biggest myth about this piece of equipment is its estimated calorie burn. Don't believe what you hear unless you are wearing a heart-rate monitor, as the numbers are drastically overblown. You can use any treadmill workout on an elliptical, adjusting your speed and the level of difficulty. I like to use the programmed workouts such as "hill" or "random." Challenge yourself with the intensity. Bring your favorite magazine or watch a TV show to make the time fly by.

Treadmill: Even if you prefer to run outside, the "dreadmill," as I often refer to it, can give you one of the highest calorie-burning workouts, thanks to its incline and variable speed ability. It can also be boring and harsh on your joints, potentially leading to injuries such as shin splints and knee pain. For this reason, I don't typically use a treadmill more than twice a week. It's also important to have proper running shoes. I recommend visiting a running specialty store to find a sneaker that fits your foot and matches your running gait. One thing to note about high-intensity interval workouts is that they can be hard to complete on a treadmill because it can take a few seconds to get up to a faster speed. Instead of a 20-second sprint interval, you end up doing just 10 seconds. Try any of the outdoor running workouts on a treadmill by increasing your intervals by an additional 10 seconds. The workouts in this section have already taken the delay into consideration.

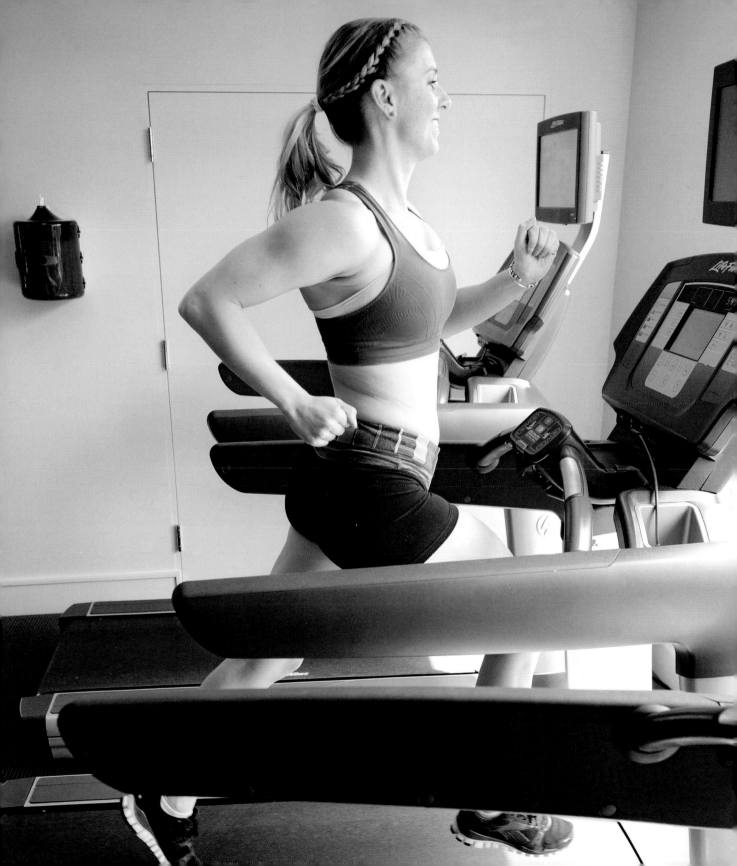

Indoor bike: This is my newest favorite piece of equipment. Spin aficionados preach the benefits of buying shoes that clip onto the pedals, but you do not need them to get a killer workout. The bike can have you breaking a sweat in less than 5 minutes. It's easy on your knees as long as you are set up properly on your bike. If you are hesitant to try a spin class, remember that the intensity depends on you! No one else can see or feel the resistance on your bike. You control the level of difficulty. Try taking a class at your local gym or studio on one of your cardio days.

Stair-climber: You have to love the machine that gives you endless stairs to help lift your booty. This machine is probably my least favorite, mainly because I find it boring. That does not mean it is not effective! Often the machines we hate are the ones that produce the best results. I encourage you to try out the stair-climber for 10 to 20 minutes while watching a favorite TV show.

The following workouts are meant to be done on a treadmill, elliptical or indoor bike. For the treadmill, use the incline and speed for directions. For the elliptical, use the rate of perceived exertion (RPE) to monitor your own intensity. The easiest rate is 1; a 10 should be an all-out effort that you can barely maintain for more than 10 seconds. For the bike, increase the speed of your legs or the resistance for the challenging intervals. Looking for a greater challenge? Increase both speed and resistance.

GYM CARDIO OPTION 1: SPEEDY INTERVAL WORKOUT

This workout is great to do on a treadmill in the morning for a 30-minute energetic start to your day. It starts slowly and allows your body to warm up. As the intensity heats up, the intervals get shorter. The pyramid style allows you to cool down gradually. Don't be afraid of the faster intervals, and feel free to go even faster once you master the workout. If you think I'm obsessed with intervals at this point, you are right! Intervals are the most efficient way to burn fat during a workout. Not only do they burn more calories during the act, but they also torch more throughout the day.

MINUTES	DURATION	INCLINE	SPEED	RPE (5–10)
0–5	5 mins	1	5.5	5 Warm-up
5–8	3 mins	2	6.5	7 Moderate
8–11	3 mins	2	5.5	6 Steady
11–13	2 mins	2	7	7 Moderate
13–15	2 mins	2	5.5	6 Steady
15–16	1 min	2	7.5	8 Difficult
16–17	1 min	2	5.5	7 Moderate
17–17:40	40 secs	2	8	9 Most Difficult
17:40–19	1 min 20 secs	2	5.5	7 Moderate
19–20	1 min	2	7.5	9 Most Difficult
20–21	1 min	2	5.5	7 Steady
21–22	1 min	2	7	8 Difficult
22–24	2 mins	2	5.5	6 Steady
24–26	2 mins	2	6.5	7 Moderate
26–28	2 mins	1	5.5	6 Steady
28–31	3 mins	1	3.5	5 Cool down

During the steady and moderate intervals, try to catch your breath as much as you can. Take advantage of your recovery periods. During the challenging faster intervals, push yourself. If you think you can run faster, try it! This workout will go by faster than you think.

GYM CARDIO OPTION 2: INTERVAL LADDER WORKOUT

Some days, I just don't feel like working out. Then, once I start, I do not want to stop! This is one of those workouts. Afterward, I always find that I have more energy left over than I thought possible. The quick intervals are great for building speed and burning fat. I love variety, so it's fun for me to switch up my routines regularly.

MINUTES	DURATION	INCLINE	SPEED	RPE (5–10)
0–5	5 mins	2	5.5	5 Warm-up
5–6	1 min	4	6	7
6–8	2 mins	4	4.0	6
8–9	1 min	5	6.5	7
9–11	2 mins	5	4.0	6
11–12	1 min	6	7.0	8
12–14	2 mins	6	4.0	6
14–15	1 min	7	7.5	8
15–17	2 mins	7	4.0	6
17–18	1 min	2	8	9
18–20	2 mins	2	4.0	6
20–21	1 min	2	8.5	9
21–23	2 mins	2	4.0	7
23–25	2 mins	2	9	10
25–30	5 mins	2	4.0	5

Have energy left in the tank? At the end of this workout, increase the incline to 8 and walk at a speed of 4.0 for an additional 5–10 minutes.

GYM CARDIO OPTION 3: FLAT INTERVALS

MINUTES	DURATION	INCLINE	SPEED	RPE (5-10)
0-5	5 mins	2	5.5	5 Warm-up
5-5:30	30 secs	2	7.5	7
5:30-7	90 secs	2	6	6
7-7:30	30 secs	2	7.5	8
7:30-9	90 secs	2	6	6
9-10:30	90 secs	2	7.5	8
10:30-11	30 secs	2	6	6
11-14	3 mins	2	4-5.5	5
Repeat everything but the 5-minute warm-up 2 more times.				

AT-THE-GYM STRETCH SEQUENCE

This sequence can be done on its own on your active rest day, or before or after a workout (or both). At a minimum, do the stretching sequence at least once a week in its entirety. To alleviate soreness from your strength training workouts, do the sequence after each strength session.

Foam rolling, also known as myofascial release, was first used by physical therapists as a means to rehab injuries and prevent them from reoccurring. Why should you use a foam roller? Because it helps reduce soreness, increases flexibility and range of motion and helps prevent getting injured in the first place. Foam rolling helps increase the flexibility of fascia, connective tissue that surrounds muscles, joints and bones. It can become too tight from overuse, which may lead to pain and even injuries. As we have become more active over the past 20 years, the use of foam rollers has expanded to the average gym goer's routine. It's a cheap way to treat yourself to a weekly sports massage. Most gyms have them. If yours does not, ask to speak with the manager about getting one.

The following routine is recommended at least once a week. If you have the time, try doing it after each strength-training session. If you don't have time, set aside 10 to 20 minutes on your active rest day to fit it in. This sequence may be a little painful at first, but if you're doing it right, the pain will go away within a week or two with regular practice. When doing the foam-rolling exercises, once you find the "hot spot," sit and breathe into it for 30 seconds. Then roll up and down the hot spot a few times to see if there is another location that needs attention. After hitting all the hot spots for a few deep breaths, move on to the next muscle group.

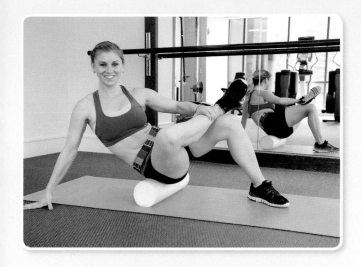

Piriformis Foam Roll: Sit down on the foam roller so that it is directly underneath your buttocks. Take your right foot and place it on your left knee. Slightly roll your hips to the right as you place your right hand behind the foam roller on the ground. Roll around the side of your glute until you feel a "hot spot," that is, where it feels like there is pressure. It should be about 3–6 inches/8–15 cm under your hip bone, on the side and toward the back of your glute. Your piriformis is small gluteal muscle that if tight can cause pain in the hips and lower back.

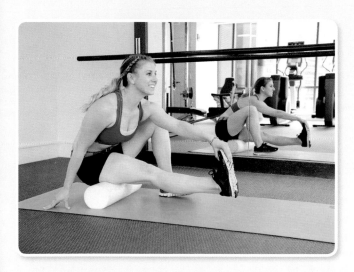

Hamstring Foam Roll: Place a foam roller directly underneath your legs where your hamstrings and glutes meet. Place your left foot on the floor and reach for your right foot with your right hand. If you can, grab hold of your toes. With your left hand on the ground behind the foam roller, massage of the back of your right thigh with the foam roller. You may need your left foot to help you balance and to let the foam roller travel. Once you find a tender spot, let the foam roller sit for 30 seconds and then find another spot. Switch legs after about 1 minute.

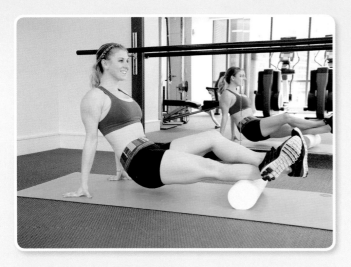

Calf Foam Roll: Position the foam roller underneath the widest part of your calves. Cross your feet so that your top calf is resting on the bottom shin. With your hands behind the foam roller, lift your hips up slightly and massage the back of your calf against the foam roller. Once you find a tender spot, let the foam roller sit for 30 seconds and then find another spot. Switch the way in which your legs are crossed after about 1 minute.

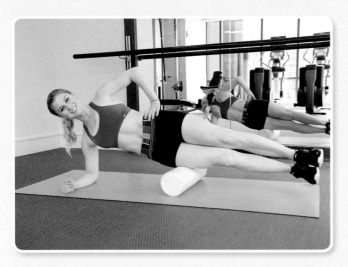

IT Band Foam Roll: Get into a side-plank forearm position with your elbow bent directly underneath your shoulder and your forearm on the floor. Place a foam roller so that it runs perpendicular to your thighs, halfway between your hip and your knee. Your feet should be lifted off the ground. Using your upper body, allow the foam roller to travel up toward your hip and then down almost to the knee. This may be painful at first. If you need to, place your top foot on the ground in front of the bottom leg that is lifted. Roll the entire IT band for an amazing stretch that will help prevent pain in your knees if you are a runner. Your IT band, the iliotibial band, is a connective tissue that runs along the outside of your thigh from the pelvis to the shin. If it gets too tight, it will cause knee pain or sometimes lead to injury in runners. To prevent this from happening, keep the IT band flexible by using a foam roller.

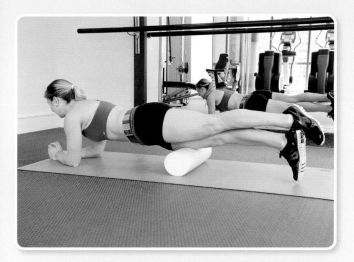

Quadriceps Foam Roll: Get into a side plank and place a foam roller underneath your thighs. Using your upper body, bring your torso forward and backward, massaging your thighs. If you do not feel anything, you may want to cross your feet and place most of your weight on one thigh. Repeat on the opposite side.

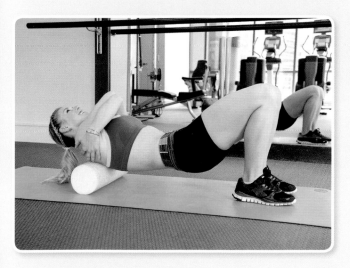

Upper Back Foam Roll: Lie down faceup with the foam roller underneath your back, just below your ribcage with arms folded across your chest, holding onto opposite shoulders. Bend your knees and bring your feet close to your butt, which should be lifted off the ground. Round your back and walk your feet out a few inches as the foam roller massages your spine toward the nape of your neck. Remember, if you find a tender spot, just hold still for 30 seconds. Bring the foam roller back down toward your mid-back by walking your feet closer to your butt. Keep rounding your back into the foam roller. Feel free to massage up and down your spine a few times, pressing your shoulder blades away from each other.

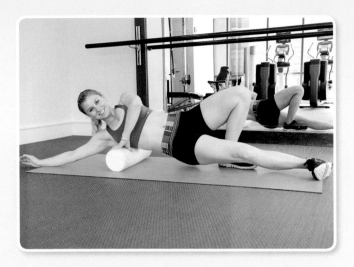

Lat Foam Roll: Lie down on the ground on your side and place the foam roller underneath your shoulder blades on the outer edge of your back. Fully extend your bottom arm and bend your top leg. Place your top foot on the ground behind the extended bottom leg. Roll up and down the outer edge of your back. Switch sides and repeat. You can also do this move with a small ball, like a tennis ball or softball.

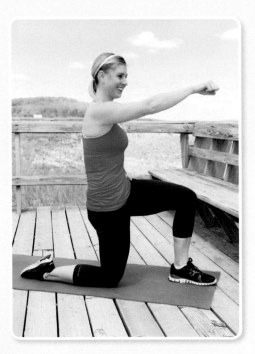

Hip Flexors Stretch: Kneel down on the ground and place your right foot out in front with your knee bent at a 90-degree angle. Extend your left arm out in front of you at shoulder height. Press your left hip forward, feeling a stretch down the left inner thigh and all the way up toward the groin area. This is one of my favorite stretches and a must after most workouts. Just sit tight and hold the stretch. It should feel amazing. Repeat on the opposite side.

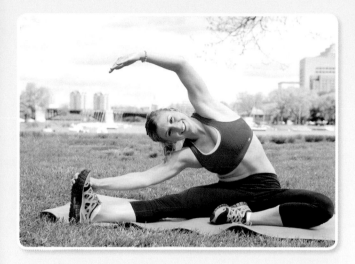

Inner Thigh Stretch: Sit down on the ground with your legs stretched out wide apart. Bend your left leg and bring your left foot in to touch the inner right thigh, just above the right knee. Reach your right arm up and over toward your right foot as your chest rotates up toward the sky, staying open. Then rotate your chest down toward the right leg and reach both arms toward your right foot. Bring your chest to your left knee. Repeat on the opposite side.

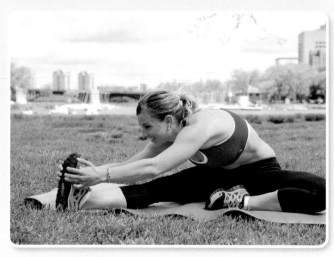

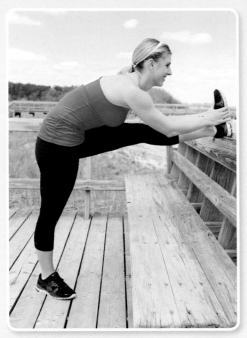

Hamstring Stretch: Stand 2 feet/61 cm away from a bar or railing that is about hip height. Lift your left leg and place your foot on top of the bar or railing. Bend forward at the hips, bringing your chest to your thigh if you can and reaching your hands toward your left foot. Feel a stretch all along the back of your hamstring. Make sure foot is relaxed and softly flexed. Switch sides and repeat.

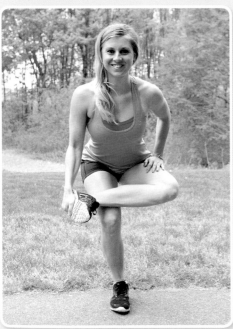

Figure-Four Stretch: Balance on your right foot. Lift your left foot and cross it over your right leg, just above the knee. Press your left knee down toward the ground to feel a stretch along the side of your glutes. Extend your hands above your head with your biceps by your ears or hold onto something at shoulder height. Try to keep your chest open and your back straight. Switch sides and repeat.

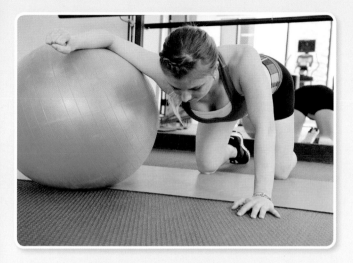

Physioball Chest Stretch: Start on all fours. With a physioball immediately to your right, place your right elbow on top of the ball, opening up the right side of your chest. Press your right shoulder gently down toward the ground to feel a stretch across your chest. Hold the position for 20–30 seconds and then switch sides and repeat.

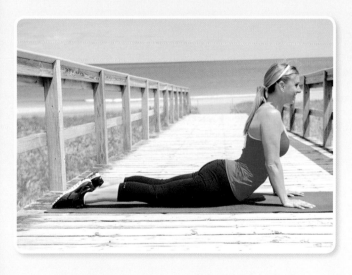

Updog: Lie facedown on the ground. Place your hands a few inches in front of your shoulders. Inhale deeply and then and as you exhale, lift your chest up off the ground, looking just a few inches in front of your hands. Use your hands to pull your torso forward slightly. Feel a gentle stretch in the lower back. Hold for a breath or two and then lower. Do 2–3 gentle lifts.

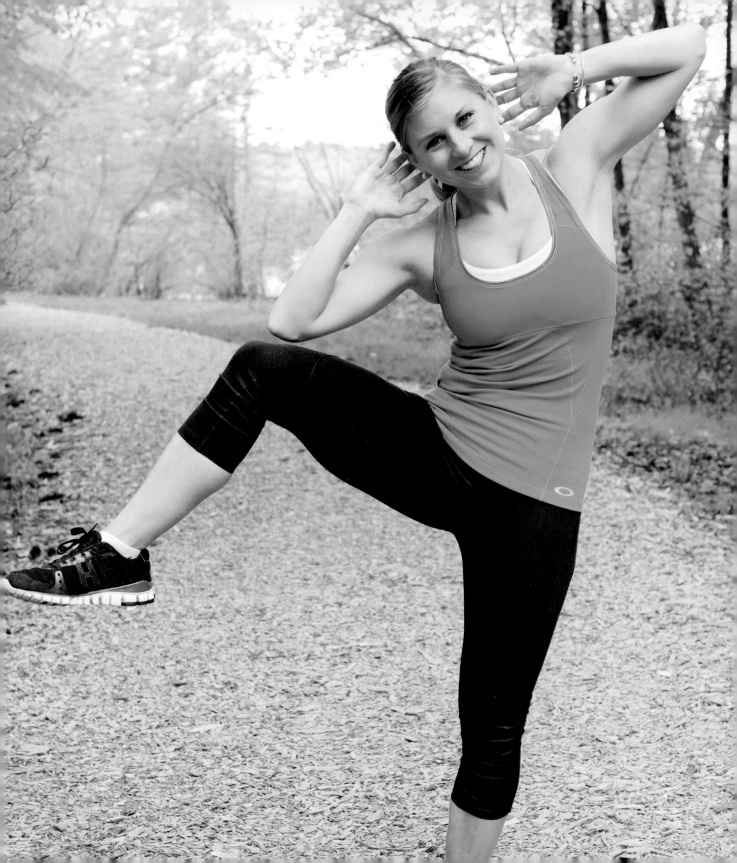

CHAPTER 3

TIME TO SPARE 10 MINUTES

Studies have shown that doing as little as 4 minutes of high-intensity work a day can be beneficial to your health. If you want to lose weight or add definition, my experience has been that 10 minutes a day is the minimum. If all you have is 4 minutes, though, that's better than nothing at all.

Though you cannot spot-reduce, causing fat to melt off specific areas of your body, you can selectively choose which body parts to focus your training on so that when the weight does come off, you have amazingly toned assets to flaunt! This chapter includes 5 different workouts that are geared toward specific goals: losing weight, flattening your abs, lifting your butt, getting rid of love handles and toning up your arms. Use these routines on their own on busy days or in addition to your scheduled full workout.

On your workout calendar, there are days dedicated to cardio and days dedicated to strength training. You can use these in workouts in two ways:

Option 1: Go ahead and do one of these routines *in addition to* your full-length workout, as prescribed in chapters 1 and 2, before or after for extra work on your trouble zone. For example, you did the Gym Strength Training Workout 2 and want more core work, so you opt to do the 10-minute ab-flattening series. If you want a double dose of cardio, try the "Goal: Lose Weight" routine first thing when you wake up and then one of the outdoor running interval workouts in the evening.

Option 2: If you can fit in only a 10-minute workout on a day dedicated to cardio, try the "Goal: Lose Weight" routine. If you can't fit in one of the strength-training routines that typically take 45 minutes to an hour to complete, do 1, 2 or 3 of the body part–specific routines to accommodate your schedule.

Do not, however, get into a routine of skipping the full-length workouts and substituting these quick 10-minute routines. You may develop muscle imbalances and could injure yourself if you do this. Some require equipment that you will need at home or at the gym.

GOAL: LOSE WEIGHT

To lose unwanted pounds, you need to eat a clean diet (which you will learn about in chapter 4) and exercise, obviously! Cardio has been shown to be more effective in burning fat than strength-training exercises. If your goal is purely to lose weight and you have only 10 minutes in your day to work out, try this routine, which is my favorite workout. The warm-up and cooldown are included in the workout.

MOVE 1:	Jog in Place, 45 seconds
MOVE 2:	Reverse Lunges with Arm Reach, 45 seconds
MOVE 3:	Forward Leg-Lift Toe Taps, 45 seconds
MOVE 4:	Side Lunge Relevés, 45 seconds
MOVE 5:	High Knees, 20 seconds
Rest, 10 seconds	
MOVE 6:	Froggers, 20 seconds
Rest, 10 seconds	
MOVE 7:	Happy Baby Dance, 20 seconds
Rest, 10 seconds	
MOVE 8:	Mountain Climbers, 20 seconds
Rest, 10 seconds	
Repeat Move 5 through Move 8, including rests	
MOVE 1:	Jog in Place, 45 seconds
MOVE 2:	Reverse Lunge with Arm Reach, 45 seconds
MOVE 3:	Forward Leg-Lift Toe Taps, 45 seconds
MOVE 4:	Side Lunge Relevés, 45 seconds

MOVE 1: **JOG IN PLACE**

Jog in place to warm up the body. Pump your arms as you lift your knees.

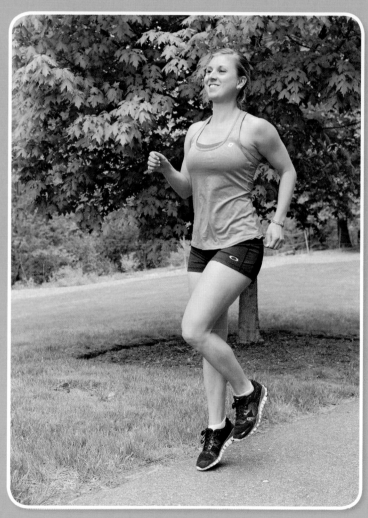

↑ **1.** Jog in place for a 45-second warm up.

MOVE 2: **REVERSE LUNGES WITH ARM REACH**

Stand with feet 1 foot/30 cm apart, hands at your sides. Step back with your left foot until your right knee forms a right angle. Lift your left arm up toward the sky and slightly over to the right. Return to the starting position and repeat with the opposite leg and arm.

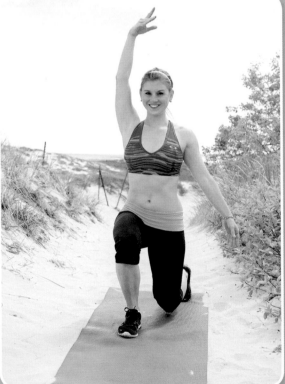

↓ 2. Step back with your left foot until your right knee forms a right angle. Lift your left arm up and slightly over to the right.

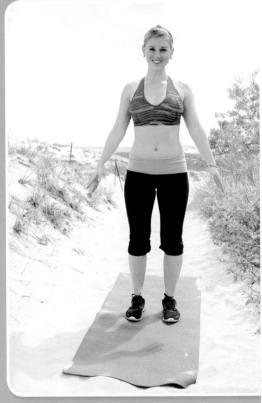

↑ 1. Stand tall with feet 1 foot apart and your hands at your sides.

MOVE 3: **FORWARD LEG-LIFT TOE TAPS**

Extend your arms straight overhead and stand tall with legs straight and feet hip distance apart. Fold at the waist as you lift one leg up at a time reaching your hands toward your foot, tapping your toe. Return to the starting position and repeat on the opposite side.

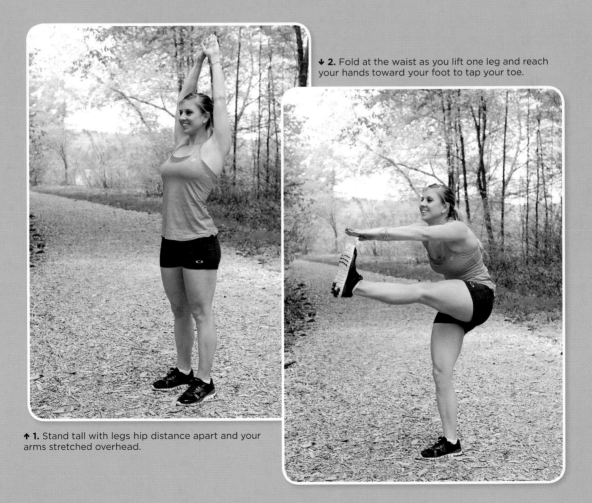

↓ 2. Fold at the waist as you lift one leg and reach your hands toward your foot to tap your toe.

↑ 1. Stand tall with legs hip distance apart and your arms stretched overhead.

MOVE 4: **SIDE LUNGE RELEVÉS**

Standing tall, balance on your tip toes, lift your arms up overhead with feet together. Bring your hands together in front of your chest while you take a large step to the left pressing your hips back and bending your knee so that your knee lines up with your ankle. With your right leg still straight, press off with the left foot to return to the starting position. Repeat on the opposite side.

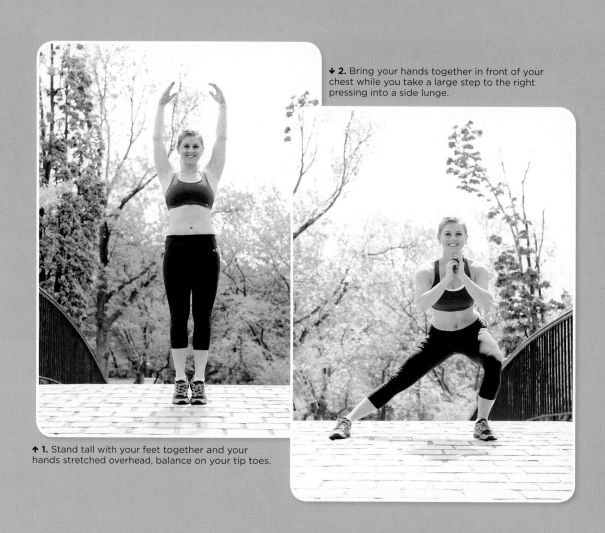

↓ **2.** Bring your hands together in front of your chest while you take a large step to the right pressing into a side lunge.

↑ **1.** Stand tall with your feet together and your hands stretched overhead, balance on your tip toes.

MOVE 5: **HIGH KNEES**

Start in a ready upright position. Begin to pump your arms while bringing your knees up as high as you can and as quickly as possible.

TIP: Since this interval is only 20 seconds long, go as hard as you can right away. Do not hold back. The benefits of high-intensity intervals are reaped only when you go all out!

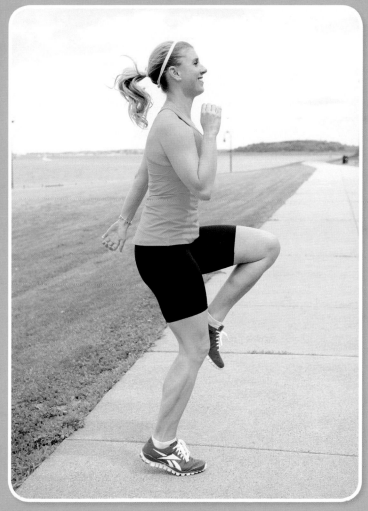

↑ **1.** Pump your arms while bringing your knees up as high as you can.

MOVE 6: **FROGGERS**

Get down on the ground and begin in a high-plank position. Jump, pulling your feet towards your hands. Land your feet on the outsides of your hands, keeping your hips low. Repeat as quickly as possible.

TIP: Try to keep your hips low for an added challenge.

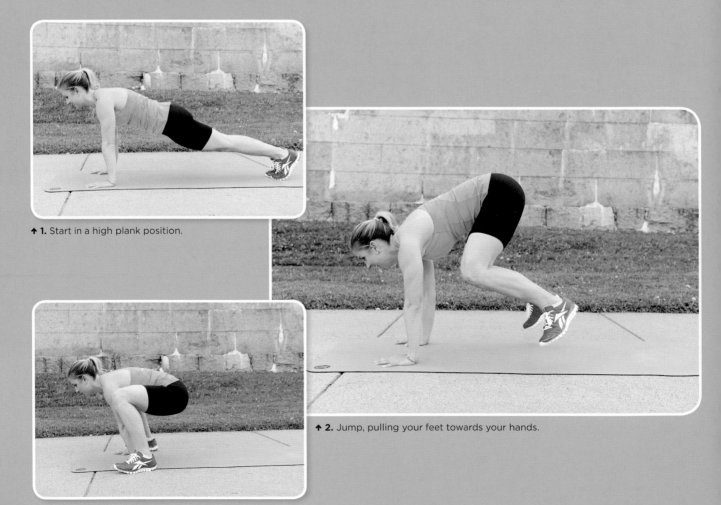

↑ **1.** Start in a high plank position.

↑ **2.** Jump, pulling your feet towards your hands.

↑ **3.** Land with your feet on the outsides of your hands, keeping your hips low.

MOVE 7: **HAPPY BABY DANCE**

Bring your hands behind your ears while standing up tall. Lift your right knee out to the side and toward your right armpit. Crunch your right elbow down toward your right knee. Hop onto your right foot and bring your left elbow toward your left knee. Quickly alternate, bringing first the right and then your left knee in toward your elbows.

TIP: This is going to be challenging, but remember that you get a 10-second rest coming up and this whole workout lasts only 10 minutes.

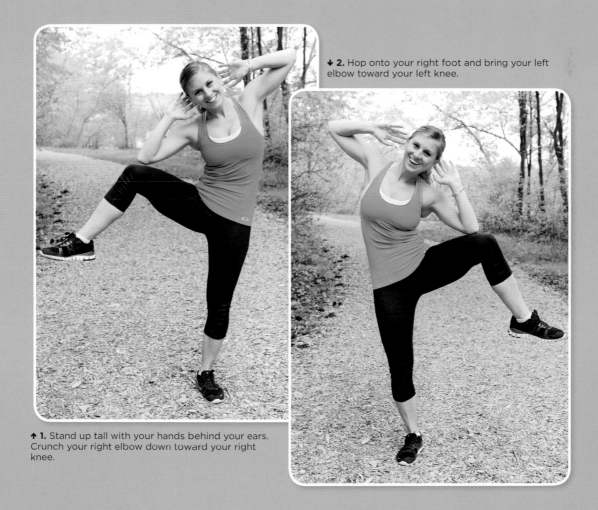

↓ **2.** Hop onto your right foot and bring your left elbow toward your left knee.

↑ **1.** Stand up tall with your hands behind your ears. Crunch your right elbow down toward your right knee.

MOVE 8: **MOUNTAIN CLIMBERS**

Begin in high-plank position, your hands underneath your shoulders, your core tight and your body forming a straight line from shoulders to ankles. Quickly alternate bringing your right knee and then your left into your chest, changing feet in midair.

TIP: Keep your back straight during this exercise. Do not let your hips hike up toward the sky. To make this move easier, bring one foot into your chest and return to the starting position before bringing the other foot to your chest.

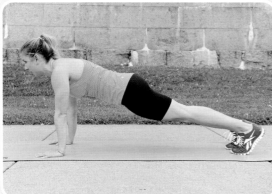

↑ **1.** Start in high-plank position.

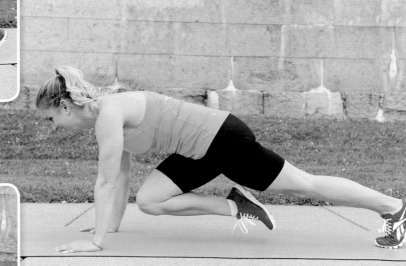

↑ **2.** Quickly alternate bringing your right knee and then your left into your chest, changing feet in midair.

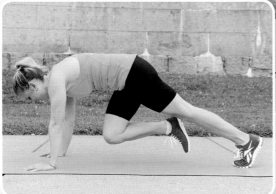

↑ **BAD:** Don't let your hips pop up. Keep your back straight.

GOAL: FLAT ABS

Abs videos on YouTube are the most popular fitness videos. Fitness alone will not get you a flat stomach. In fact, abs are made in the kitchen! Abdominal exercises will strengthen your core and help you stand up straight, making you look leaner without losing a single pound. They will also help create definition that will be visible when you lose most of your excess abdominal fat.

If you are reading this and thinking, "I want flat abs now," I suggest you focus first on your diet. Doing this routine in addition to your workout and clean diet is a great way to see quicker results. If you have only 2 minutes for your core, do a plank. It's my favorite move for my midsection because it yields results quickly, and there is minimal risk of injury or of doing it incorrectly. If you cannot hold a plank for a full minute, hold it for as long as you can. When it comes time to drop down to your knees, lower for 5 seconds and then lift back up. Hold for another 5–10 seconds. Rest for 5 and hold again. Continue until you reach 1 minute. If 1 minute becomes too easy, amp it up to 90 seconds! If you have 10 minutes, do this routine. It's sure to tone, strengthen and sculpt your core.

MOVE 1:	Forearm Plank, 1 minute
MOVE 2:	Toe Touches, 20 reps
MOVE 3:	Physioball Jacknifes, 20 reps
MOVE 4:	Shin Slaps, 10 each side
MOVE 5:	Physioball Pikes (use paper towels, disc or ball), 10 reps
MOVE 1:	Forearm Plank, 1 minute
MOVE 6:	Teasers, 8
MOVE 7:	Scissors, 20 crisscrosses

MOVE 1: **FOREARM PLANK**

Lie down on your stomach and place your elbows directly underneath your shoulders, with forearms pressed into the ground. Make fists with both hands or clasp them together. Tuck your toes underneath. Lift your knees off the ground and form a straight line from your shoulders to your ankles. Squeeze your glutes, press your shoulders down and away from your ears while pinching your shoulder blades together. Keep your belly sucked in as if someone were about to punch you in the gut.

TIP: For an advanced plank, lift one leg up in the air. After 30 seconds, lift the opposite leg for the same amount of time.

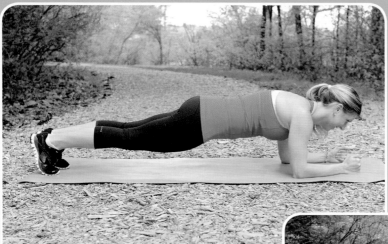

↑ 1. Start in plank position, resting on your forearms.

↓ ADVANCED: For an advanced plank, alternate holding each leg up in the air.

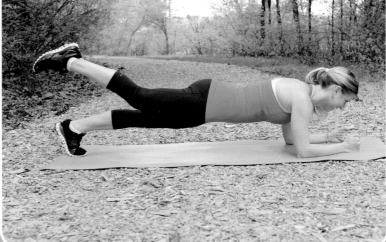

MOVE 2: TOE TOUCHES

Lie down on your back with your feet together, legs straight in the air and your hands held up toward your toes. Lift your torso and shoulder blades up off the ground and reach up for your toes. Lower your torso and repeat.

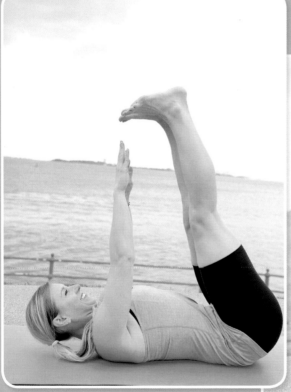

↑ **1.** Lie down on your back with your feet together, legs straight in the air and your hands held up toward your toes.

↓ **2.** Lift your torso and shoulder blades up off the ground and reach up for your toes.

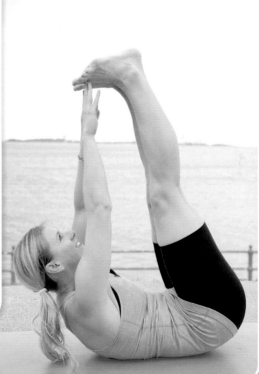

MOVE 3: **PHYSIOBALL JACKKNIFES**

Place the tops of your feet on a physioball and walk your hands out until you are balancing in a high-plank position with your feet on top of the ball. Exhale and bring both knees in toward your chest, keeping the tops of your feet balanced on top of the ball. Slowly straighten your legs back to return to high-plank position.

TIP: Do not let your hips rise up too high when you bring the ball in toward your chest. As you return to the starting position, don't let your hips sink, either.

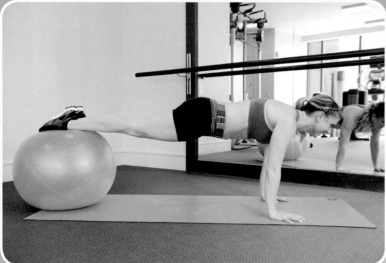

↑ **1.** Place the tops of your feet on a physioball and walk your hands out until you are balancing in a high-plank position.

↓ **2.** Bring both knees in toward your chest, keeping the tops of your feet balanced on top of the ball.

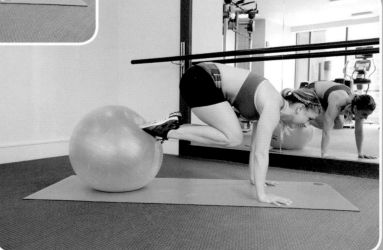

MOVE 4: **SHIN SLAPS**

Lie down on your back with your legs shoulder width apart and your arms extended at your sides. Raise your left arm up and raise right leg at the same time. Reach your left hand to your right shin. Lower your arm and leg and repeat on the opposite side, reaching your right hand to your left shin.

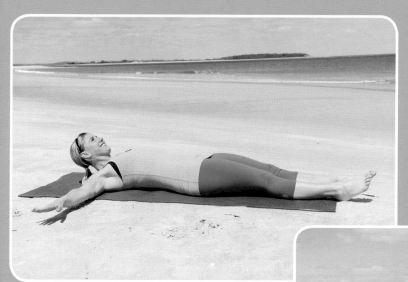

↓ 2. Raise your left arm up as you raise your right leg and touch your left shin with your right hand.

↑ 1. Lie down on your back with your legs shoulder width apart and your arms extended at your sides.

MOVE 5: **PHYSIOBALL PIKES**

Start in a high-plank position with your feet on top of a physioball, hands underneath shoulders. Engage your core and hinge at the hips, lifting them up toward the sky, keeping your legs straight as you bring the ball in toward your hands. You can lift your hips up as high as they can go or until they are in line with your shoulders and you form a straight line from your hands to your tailbone. Your head is below your heart and hips. Keep your legs straight as you lower to the starting position.

TIP: Don't have a physioball? Do this move with a sliding disc or paper plate on hardwood floors.

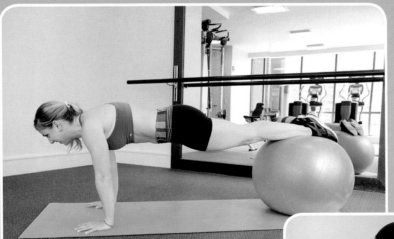

↓ 2. Hinge at the hips, lifting them up toward the sky, keeping your legs straight as you bring the ball in toward your hands.

↑ 1. Start in a high-plank position with your feet on top of a physioball.

MOVE 6: **TEASERS**

Start lying face-up on the ground with your feet together and outstretched, your arms extending overhead. Inhale and as you exhale, rise up into a V position with your hands reaching toward your toes, your arms and legs straight. Your legs should come to a 45-degree angle to your torso.

TIP: If you are a beginner, bend your legs at the knees to a 90-degree angle when you raise your torso and head.

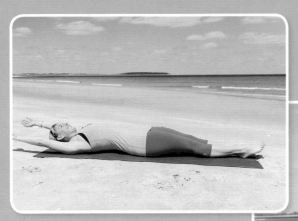

↑ **1.** Start lying face-up on the ground with your feet together and outstretched, your arms extending overhead.

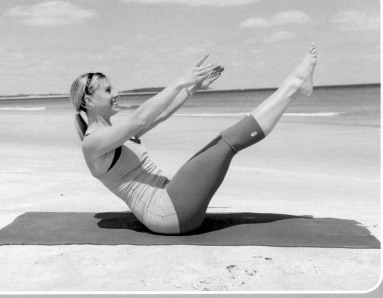

↑ **2.** Rise up into a V position with your hands reaching toward your toes.

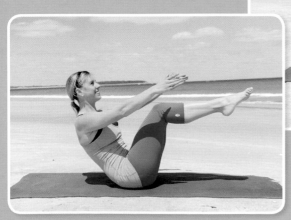

↑ **3.** If you're a beginner, bend your legs at the knees to a 90-degree angle when you raise your torso and head.

MOVE 7: SCISSORS

Lie down on your back with your hands under your butt, your feet together off the floor at a 45-degree angle or lower. Begin to cross your feet, one on top of the other, in a crisscross motion. Your legs should be long and straight. Press your navel into your lower back.

TIP: Do not let your back arch up away from the ground. If it begins to lift up, raise your legs closer to a 90-degree angle.

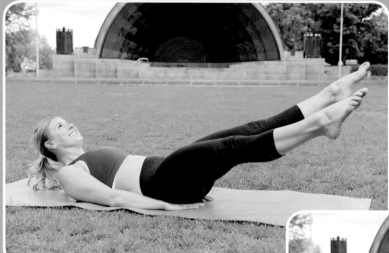

↓ 2. Cross your feet, one on top of the other, in a crisscross motion.

↑ 1. Lie down on your back with your hands under your butt, your feet together off the floor at a 45-degree angle or lower.

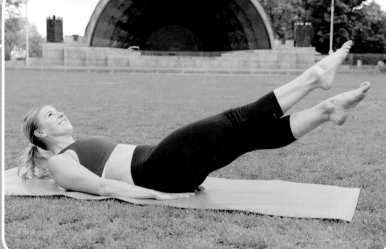

GOAL: LIFT YOUR BUTT

Genetics play a big part in your body shape, especially your booty. You will never look like Kim Kardashian from doing lunges or squats. Some women just have big booties. Neither Jennifer Lopez nor Beyoncé will ever look like Kelly Ripa, and vice versa. The size of your backside may be difficult to control, but you can lift and tone it with these simple, tried-and-true exercises. These are my favorite moves when it comes to looking good in a bikini from behind. They focus exclusively on lifting and toning your booty by working the gluteus maximus, gluteus medius and hamstrings.

MOVE 1:	Single-Leg Hip Lifts, 15 reps on the left
MOVE 2:	Weighted Donkey Kicks (5-8 lb/2-3.5 kg dumbbell), 15 reps on the left
MOVE 1:	Single-Leg Hip Lifts, 15 reps on the right
MOVE 2:	Weighted Donkey Kicks (5-8 lb/2-3.5 kg dumbbell), 15 reps on the right
MOVE 3:	Single-Leg Squats, 12 reps on the left
MOVE 3:	Single-Leg Squats, 12 reps on the right
MOVE 4:	Hamstring Curls with Exercise Ball , 15 reps
MOVE 5:	Sumo Squat Series, 20 reps
Repeat the sequence from the top for a total of two sets.	

GOAL: LIFT YOUR BUTT

MOVE 1: SINGLE-LEG HIP LIFTS

Lie on your back with your left foot flexed and extended straight up toward the ceiling. Your right leg should be bent with your foot on the floor, heel close to your butt. Arms should be extended by your sides, your palms facing down. Press through your right heel and lift your hips off the ground, squeezing your left glute. Your right leg should not move and your hips should stay level. Rise only as high as you can go without arching your back. Lower your butt until it grazes the ground and lift it right back up. Do 15 reps on the left leg before moving onto the Weighted Donkey Kick.

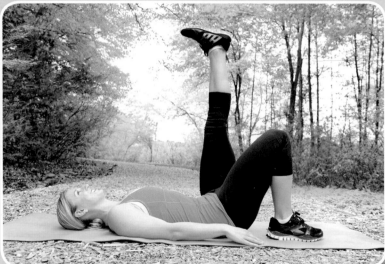

↑ 1. Lie on your back with your left foot extended straight up toward the ceiling and left leg bent with your foot on the floor.

↓ 2. Press through your right heel and lift your hips off the ground.

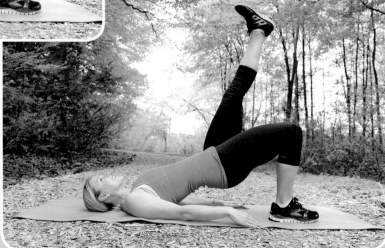

MOVE 2: **WEIGHTED DONKEY KICKS**

Start on all fours with your knees directly under your hips and your hands underneath your shoulders. Place a 5-8 lb/2-3.5 kg dumbbell behind your left knee and squeeze it to hold it in place. Raise your left heel up toward the sky, keeping a slight bend in your knee and making sure the dumbbell does not fall out. Keep your core engaged and hips tucked under so that your hip bones are curling up toward your shoulders. Lower the leg back down slowly. Do 15 reps on the left side before doing the Single-Leg Hip Lift on the right side, followed by the Weighted Donkey Kick on the right.

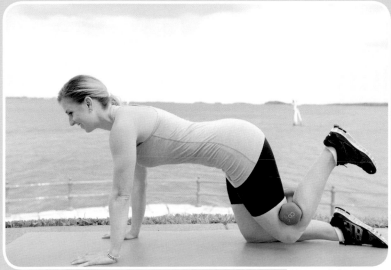

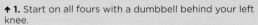
↑ **1.** Start on all fours with a dumbbell behind your left knee.

↓ **2.** Raise your left heel up toward the sky, keeping a slight bend in your knee and making sure the dumbbell does not fall out.

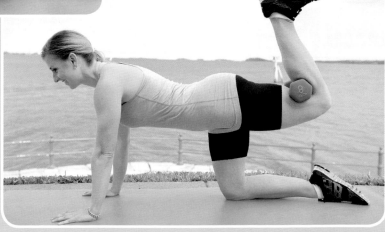

MOVE 3: **SINGLE-LEG SQUATS**

Stand up tall with your arms bent and your fists in front of your chest. Raise one foot slightly in front of your torso and balance on the other. Lower yourself into a squat on one foot, keeping your knee stable, until your thigh is almost parallel with the ground. Press up through your heel, slowly returning to the starting position. Remember to keep your chest open and your eyes forward.

TIP: To make this move harder, lower yourself until your butt grazes the floor and your lifted leg shoots out parallel to the ground. Keep your knee bending in the same direction that your toes are pointing. Make this move easier by placing a bench behind you. Lower yourself onto the bench and rise back up pressing through the heel. This is great for beginners to get the feel of this move. It's one of my favorites!

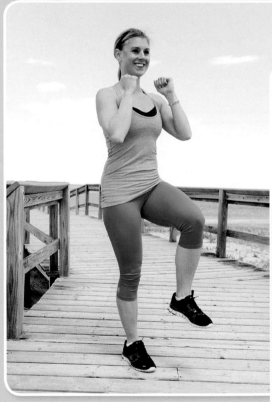

↑ 1. Stand up tall with your fists in front of your chest and one foot slightly raised.

↓ **2.** Lower yourself into a squat on one foot, keeping your knee stable.

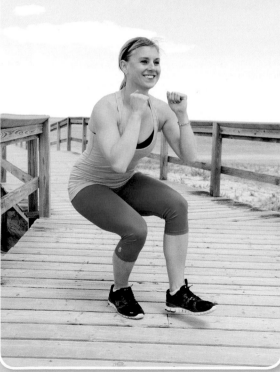

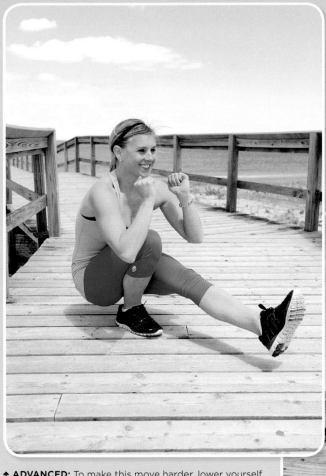

↓ BEGINNER: Make this move easier by lowering yourself onto a bench.

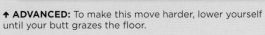

↑ ADVANCED: To make this move harder, lower yourself until your butt grazes the floor.

MOVE 4: **HAMSTRING CURLS WITH PHYSIOBALL**

Start by lying faceup on the ground. Place your feet on top of a physioball, your legs extended but slightly bent at the knee. Extend your arms along your sides, palms facing the ground. Balance by pressing your heels into the ball and flexing your feet. Lift your hips up off the ground. Curl your heels in toward your glutes as you lift your hips slightly higher than the starting position. Maintain your balance by pressing your hands into the ground. Slowly lower your heels to the starting position before repeating this move.

TIP: To make this move more difficult, try lifting one leg up toward the ceiling and curling in one leg at a time on top of the physioball for an added glute burn.

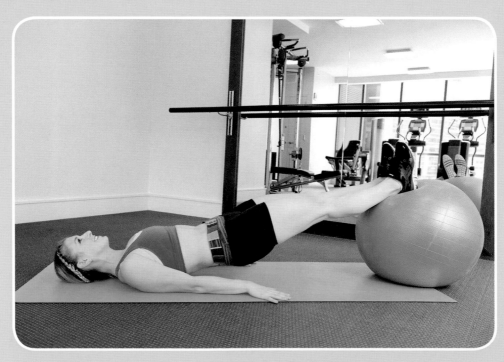

↑ **1.** Start by lying face-up on the ground with your feet on top of a physioball.

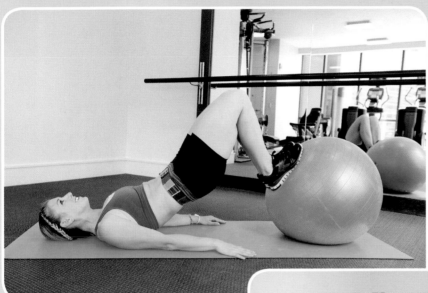

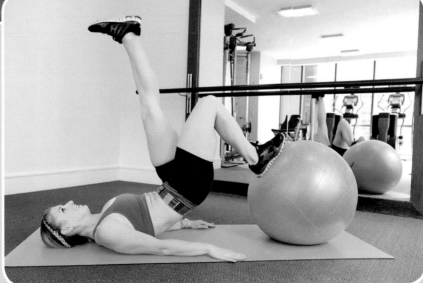

3. To make this move more difficult, try lifting one leg at a time up toward the ceiling and curling in the opposite leg.

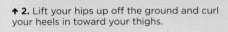

↑ **2.** Lift your hips up off the ground and curl your heels in toward your thighs.

MOVE 5: **SUMO SQUAT SERIES**

Stand with your feet wider than shoulder width apart, toes pointing forward and slightly out in the same direction as your knees. To help with balance, extend your arms out to the sides. If you have access to a bar, feel free to grab it with one hand. Lower yourself until your thighs are parallel with the ground. Press through your heels, squeezing your glutes to return to starting position and then into a lower position by about 1–2 inches/2.5–5 cm. Repeat 20 times. Next, lower yourself until your thighs are parallel with the ground, but instead of coming all the way up to standing position, come only halfway up. Slowly pulse up and down 1 inch/2.5 cm 20 times with your hips tucked and rotating up toward your rib cage. Lift up your left heel and balance on the ball of your left foot with your right foot planted firmly on the ground. Pulse gently up 1 inch/2.5 cm and down 1 inch/2.5 cm 20 times. Place your left heel back on the ground and raise the right heel up. Pulse 20 times on the left side. Lift both heels up and finish with 20 quick 1 inch/2.5 cm up and 1 inch/ 2.5 cm down pulses, balancing on the balls of both feet. Remember to keep your back straight, chest open, core engaged and, most of all, hips tucked under. Pretend you are trying to curl your hip bones up toward your collarbone. It's okay if your legs to start to shake. That means you're working hard to tighten your tush and achieve lean thighs. Make sure you stretch after this workout!

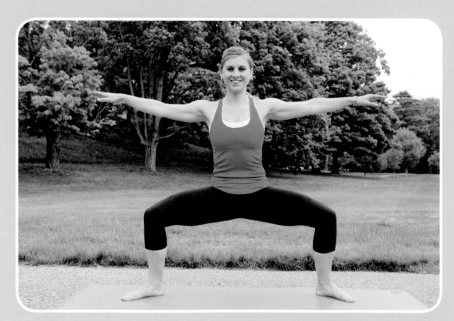

↑ 1. Stand with your feet wider than shoulder width apart and your arms extended out at your sides. Lower yourself until your thighs are parallel with the ground.

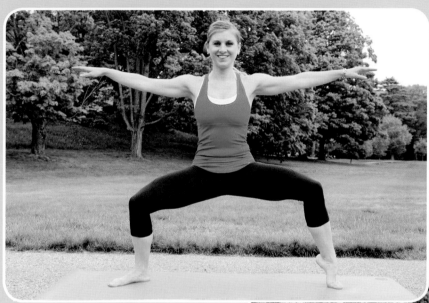

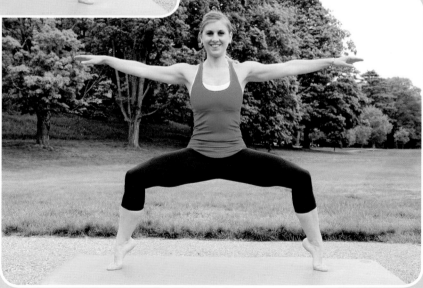

↓ 3. Lift both heels up and finish with 20 quick pulses.

↑ 2. Lift up your left heel and balance on the ball of your left foot with your right foot planted firmly on the ground. Pulse.

GOAL: GET RID OF LOVE HANDLES

If the pants you are wearing are too tight around the waist, regardless of your body fat percentage, you will look like you have "love handles." This is why even skinny celebrities wear Spanx and the founder of the shapewear company is worth a billion dollars. Once you reduce the fat around your midsection, you will be able to see the results from an obliques-focused routine like this one, as it will chisel the sides of your waist, creating sexy definition.

This routine focuses on your obliques, the muscles that run along the sides of your core. Repeat the following sequence twice without resting between sets or exercises.

MOVE 1:	Side Plank Elbow-to-Knee Kisses, 10 reps on each side
MOVE 2:	Spiderman Crunches, 10 reps on each side
MOVE 3:	Russian Twists (5-10 lb/2-5 kg dumbbell), 20 reps on each side
MOVE 4:	Dumbbell Drags (5-10 lb/2-5 kg dumbbell), 10 reps
MOVE 5:	Bicycles, 20 reps

MOVE 1: SIDE PLANK ELBOW-TO-KNEE KISSES

Begin on your right side with your right elbow on the ground, under your right shoulder, your right forearm on the ground facing forward. Stack your left foot on top of your right and left hand on your hip. Lift your hips so your body forms a straight line from your shoulders to your ankles. Extend your left arm above your head with your bicep next to your ear. Bend your left elbow and bring it toward your waist as you lift your left knee to meet it. That's one rep—now return to the starting position, stretching the side of body as long as you can, and repeat. Complete all 10 reps before switching sides.

TIP: If this is too hard, lower your right knee toward the ground.

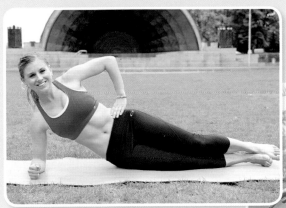

↑ **1.** Begin on your right side with your right forearm on the ground facing forward. Stack your feet and put your left hand on your hip.

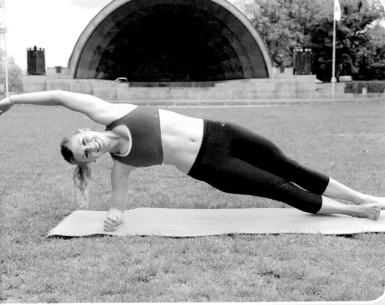

↑ **2.** Lift your hips up so that your body forms a straight line and extend your left arm above your head.

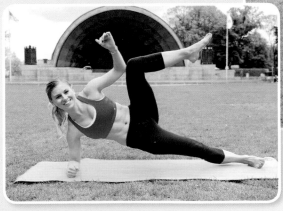

↑ **3.** Bend your left elbow and bring it toward your waist as you lift your left knee to meet it.

MOVE 2: **SPIDERMAN CRUNCHES**

Begin in high-plank position with your hands placed directly underneath shoulders and your body forming a straight line from your shoulders to your ankles. Bring your right knee to your right elbow, keeping your back straight and crunching the right side of your body, cinching at the waist. Keep your abs pulled in toward your spine. Return your right leg to the starting position and repeat on the opposite side. Do 10 crunches to alternating sides for a total of 20.

TIP: This move is a total core killer and one of my favorites. It will flatten your belly while toning your obliques.

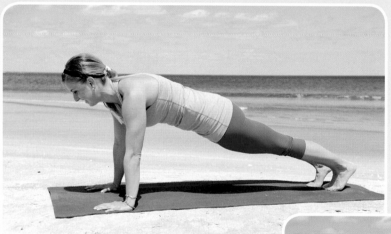

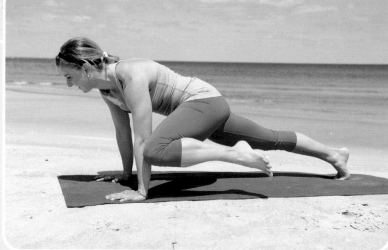

↓ 2. Bring your left knee to your left elbow, keeping your back straight and crunching the left side of your body, Alternate sides.

↑ 1. Begin in high-plank position.

MOVE 3: RUSSIAN TWISTS

Grab a weight or medicine ball (5–10 lbs/2–5 kg) if you have one available; if not, do this exercise without the weight. Start in a V-sit position with your back straight, chest open, legs together and bent with your feet off the ground. Hold the weight in front of your chest. Lower the weight to the left side, tapping it to the ground while keeping your chest facing forward. Drop your legs and lower them slightly to the right. Bring the weight back to center and then drop it to the right side, dropping your legs slightly to the left. Alternate dropping the weight to each side at a fairly quick pace. Do 20 total reps to each side. Breathe out each time you switch sides and keep your navel pulled into your lower back the entire time.

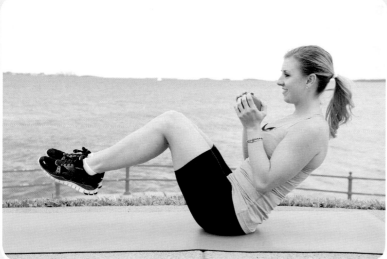

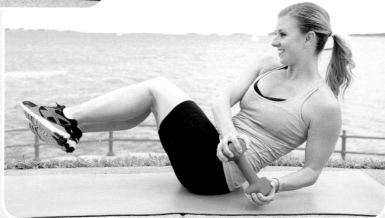

↓ 2. Lower the weight to the left side, tapping it to the ground while keeping your chest facing forward. Drop your legs and lower them slightly to the right. Alternate.

↑ 1. Hold a weight and start in a V-sit position with your back straight, chest open, legs together and bent with your feet off the ground.

MOVE 4: **DUMBBELL DRAGS**

Start in a high-plank position with your hands under your shoulders, core tight and heels pressing away from your kneecaps. Place a 5–10 lb/2–5 kg dumbbell a few inches down and to the outside of your right hand. Raise your left hand and grab the weight without rotating hips. Do not move anything else besides your left hand. Bring the dumbbell to the left side and place it a few inches past your shoulder and slightly lower than where your left hand began. Repeat with the right arm for 1 rep. Repeat for a total of 10 reps per side.

TIP: Challenge yourself to keep your hips level. Your arms should be the only body part moving, but this is a core exercise. Your abs and lower back have to work to keep the rest of your body stable.

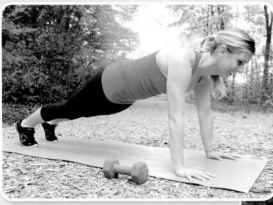

↑ **1.** Start in a high-plank position with a weight to the outside of your right hand.

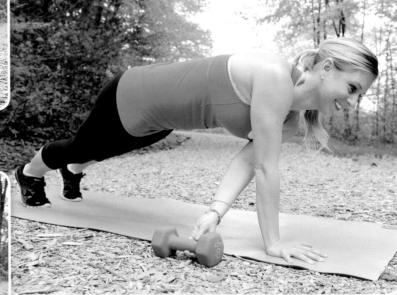

↑ **2.** Raise your left hand and grab the weight without rotating your hips. Bring the dumbbell to the left side.

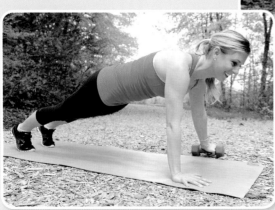

↑ **3.** Repeat with the right arm for 1 rep.

MOVE 5: **BICYCLES**

Lie on your back with your knees bent 90 degrees and your shins parallel to the floor, in a tabletop position. Your hands should be placed gently behind the your ears but not pulling on your head. Bring your right knee to your left elbow as you twist your core and fully extend your left leg, about 6–12 inches/15–30 cm above the ground. Switch sides for 1 rep.

TIP: Do this move slowly for an added challenge. Really focus on looking at your opposite elbow. If you are bringing your right elbow to your left knee, look for your left elbow behind your head for a more effective bicycle crunch.

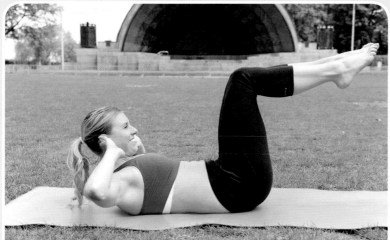

↓ 2. Bring your right knee to your left elbow as you twist your core and fully extend your left leg.

↑ 1. Lie on your back with your knees bent 90 degrees and your shins parallel to the floor. Your hands should be placed gently behind your ears.

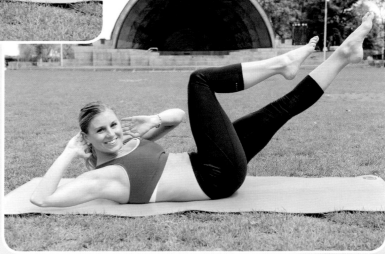

GOAL: TONE YOUR ARMS

Arms are similar to the rest of your body in that genetics play a part in how easy it may be for you to lose fat or create definition. If you put muscle on fairly easily and have an athletic build, you will be able to tone your shoulders, biceps and triceps in 2 to 4 weeks. If you have a small build with minimal muscle, you will need to work harder for similar gains. Trust me when I say (again) that you will not bulk up. As you progress, increase the weights that you are using. You may also increase the number of reps, but that will make this routine longer than 10 minutes. The idea is that you do not want to be able to handle any additional reps by the end! You will need dumbbells for this workout.

MOVE 1:	Bicep Curls to Shoulder Presses (5-15 lb/2.3-6.8 kg dumbbells), 12-15 reps
MOVE 2:	Plank Rows with T-Twists (8-20 lb/3.6-9 kg dumbbells), 8 reps
MOVE 3:	High-to-Low Planks, 8 reps
MOVE 4:	Upright Rows (5-15 lb/2.3-6.8 kg dumbbells), 12–15 reps
MOVE 5:	Triceps Dips, 20 reps
MOVE 6:	Push-Ups, as many reps as possible (AMRAP)
Repeat twice for a total of 3 sets	

MOVE 1: **BICEP CURLS TO SHOULDER PRESSES**

Suggested weight: 5–15 lb/2.3–6.8 kg dumbbells

Standing up tall, chest open, knees slightly bent and hips tucked. Hold two dumbbells in front of your thighs with your arms long and palms facing away from your body. Slowly curl the dumbbells up towards your armpits. At the top, rotate your palms to face away from your body and open your elbows out to the sides. Press the dumbbells up overhead so that they are in line with your shoulders and your arms are fully extended. Reversing your movements, slowly lower the dumbbells. Repeat. This double-duty move will tone your shoulders and biceps.

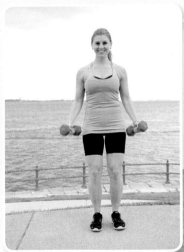

↑ **1.** Stand tall while holding two dumbbells in front of your thighs.

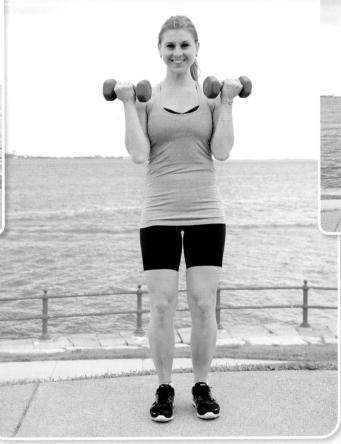

↑ **2.** Slowly curl the dumbbells up toward your armpits.

↑ **3.** Then rotate your palms to face away from you body and press the dumbbells up overhead.

MOVE 2: **PLANK ROWS WITH T-TWISTS**

Suggested weight: 8–20 lbs/3.6–9 kg dumbbells

Start in a high-plank position holding onto a set of dumbbells placed underneath your shoulders, your palms facing in. Your feet should be slightly more than shoulder width apart. Your core should be engaged, shoulder blades pressing away from each other and down away from your ears. Squeeze your glutes and lift your kneecaps toward your thighs. Keeping your hips level, bring the right dumbbell to just above your right hip, pulling directly from below your right shoulder blade. Rotate your chest to the right and extend your right arm up toward the sky with your hips stacked on top of each other. Slowly reverse your movements to return to the starting position. Repeat on the opposite side. Try not to rock from side to side.

TIP: This move works your shoulders, back and core. If it's too hard to keep your hips level during the row, widen the distance between your feet.

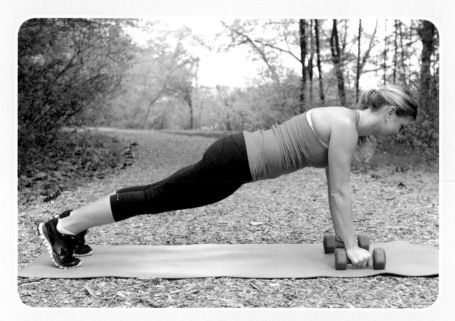

↟ **1.** Start in a high-plank position holding onto a set of dumbbells.

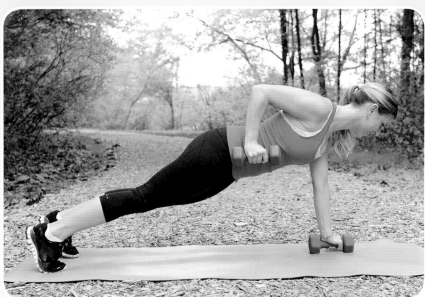

2. Bring the right dumbbell to just above your right hip, pulling directly from below your right shoulder blade.

3. Rotate your chest to the right and extend your right arm up toward the sky.

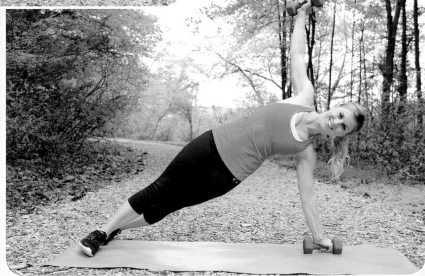

MOVE 3: **HIGH-TO-LOW PLANKS**

Start in a high-plank position with your feet hip width apart and hands underneath your shoulders. Engage your core by pulling your navel in toward your lower back. Lower yourself one arm at time onto your forearms until you are in a forearm plank. Your body should form a straight line from your shoulders to your ankles. One arm at a time, press back up.

TIP: To make this move more advanced, add a push-up before going down onto your forearms. This move will never get easy. It's a total-body-tightening exercise. Focus on really pulling your navel in toward your lower back and squeezing your glutes for extra butt and core benefits.

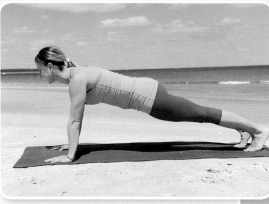

↑ **1.** Start in a high-plank position.

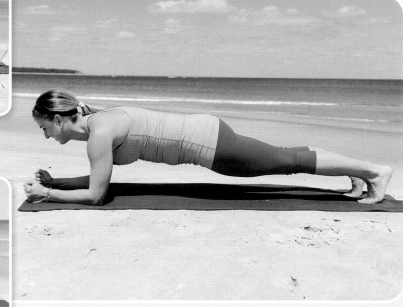

↑ **2.** Lower yourself one arm at a time onto your forearms until you are in a forearm plank.

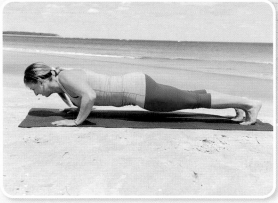

↑ **3.** To make this move more advanced, add a push-up before going down onto your forearms.

MOVE 4: **UPRIGHT ROWS**

Suggested weight: 5–15 lbs/2.3–6.8 kg dumbbells

Stand up holding on to a pair of dumbbells in front of your body with your palms facing the tops of your thighs. Slowly raise the dumbbells up toward your shoulders, your elbows out wide and the dumbbells close to your chest. Stop once your elbows are even with your shoulders and then slowly return to the starting position. This move is a favorite of mine for creating strong shoulders with sexy definition.

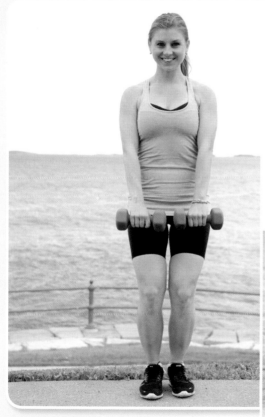

↑ **1.** Stand up holding on to a pair of dumbbells in front of your body.

↓ **2.** Slowly raise the dumbbells up toward your shoulders, your elbows out wide and the dumbbells close to your chest.

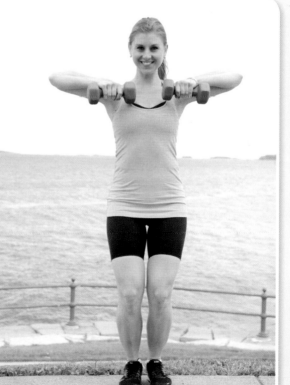

MOVE 5: **TRICEPS DIPS**

Sit on the ground with your knees bent and feet about 16 inches/40 cm away from your butt. Place your hands down on the ground a few inches behind your butt with your fingers pointing toward your feet and rotated slightly out to the side. Lift your hips up off the ground but keep your back close to your arms. Tuck your hips under. Bend your arms at the elbow to lower your hips toward the ground. Go as far down as you can without your butt touching the ground. Press through the heel of your hands to return to the starting position. You may do it on a bench if one is available.

TIP: This move works your triceps. To make this move more challenging, straighten your legs so your feet are as far away from your butt as possible while keeping your torso close to your arms. Tuck your hips up toward your shoulders to increase the amount of distance you can lower them.

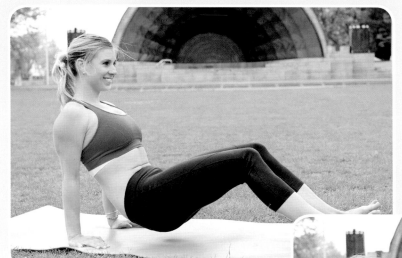

↓ 2. Bend your arms at the elbow to lower your hips toward the ground.

↑ 1. Sit on the ground with your knees bent, your hands behind your butt and your hips up off the ground.

MOVE 6: PUSH-UPS

Start in a modified position, your knees bent on the floor and hands underneath and slightly wider than shoulder distance apart. Lower yourself into a push-up, maintaining the straight line that your body has formed. Keep your chin up and look about 6 inches/15 cm in front of your hands. Press back up to the starting position. Do as many reps as you can before fatigue makes it impossible to continue.

Repeat this sequence twice for a 10-minute workout. If you have more time, feel free to do more.

TIP: Make this move harder by doing the push-ups on your toes.

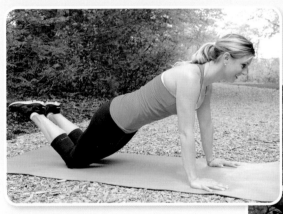

↑ **1.** Start in a modified push up position, kneeling.

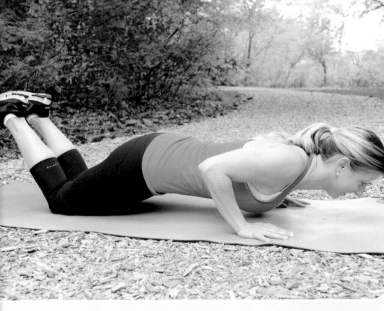

↑ **2.** Lower yourself into a push-up, maintaining the straight line that your body has formed.

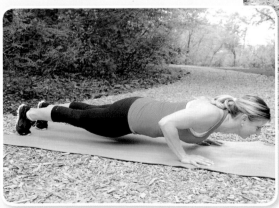

↑ **ADVANCED:** Make this move harder by doing the push-ups on your toes.

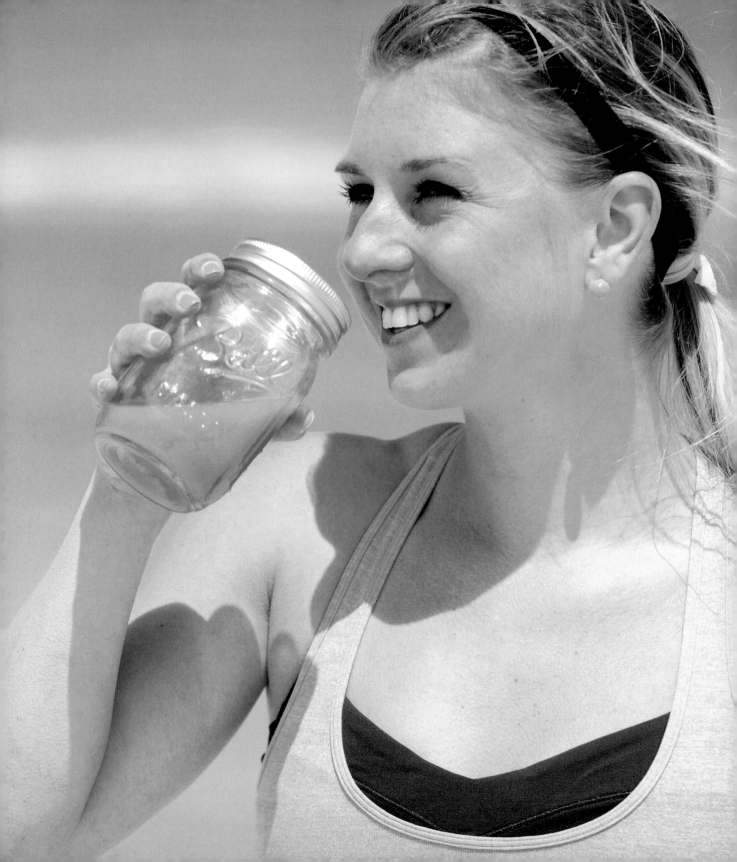

PART TWO

TIME TO
EAT CLEAN
TO GET LEAN

In my early twenties, I had a few diet books and would cut recipe ideas out of magazines. The ones that sounded the best always had a long list of ingredients with many herbs and spices. When I went to the grocery store and discovered how expensive some of the items were, I would often bail on my efforts to be the healthy version of Martha Stewart.

Though many healthy ingredients are worth the extra money, eating at home is supposed to cost less than eating out. I never understood the point of the complicated recipes in those diet books. After all, who has the time or money? And I can't stand when produce goes bad. It's like throwing dollars down the drain. Making meals to get skinny again is simple. There shouldn't be a million ingredients. The more flavors there are in a dish, studies have shown, the more likely it is that you will overeat. Of course, the food needs to taste good in order for you to want to eat it, but you also have to have the foods on hand and remember to buy what you need without relying on a list. Getting skinny again will become a reality when you learn how to grocery shop intuitively for healthy meals all week long. That is what this section is dedicated to teaching you.

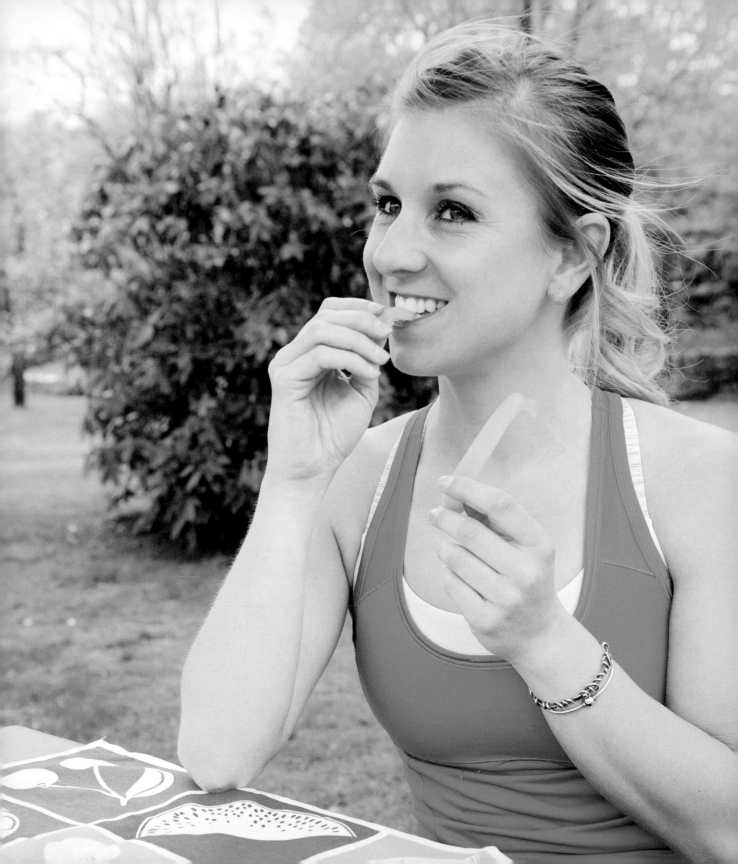

CHAPTER 4

TIME TO EAT RIGHT

Most people do not lose weight by accident. It takes a deliberate effort and self-control. Knowing what to eat and how much are the two most important rules.

This is not a diet book. Those help people lose weight temporarily. That weight almost always comes back, too! I want you to stop "crash dieting." When you restrict, you end up binging. This plan is for you to maintain a weight that you feel sexy and confident at, yet you can still indulge in the occasional cocktail or dessert. Your weight will healthily fluctuate as much as 5 pounds/ 2.3 kg up or down, but this plan is structured so that you no longer have to say, "I'm on a diet." I want you to be able to control your weight without counting every calorie.

EAT-CLEAN BASICS

Let's begin with the basics. I'm a believer in eating clean, which means avoiding processed foods and artificial ingredients and eating more fruits, vegetables, lean proteins and whole grains. You should be able to recognize most of the ingredients on your food label—if there even is one.

I believe in crowding out bad foods rather than eliminating them. Instead of saying no to ice cream after dinner, say yes to some High-Protein Banana Soft-Serve. Save the ice cream for summer vacations when you are able to indulge in homemade. one-of-a-kind flavors! Instead of swearing off sweet potato fries at a restaurant, bake your own at home. I promise, mine taste better.

Add foods to your diet that are full of nutrients so that you are full and do not crave the junk. Discover versatile new foods as well that are better alternatives to old comfort recipes—for example, swapping coconut flour for bread crumbs in meatloaf or using protein powder instead of flour in baked goods.

HOW MANY CALORIES SHOULD YOU EAT?

This depends on your sex, age, activity level, current weight, desired weight, how soon you want to achieve your goal and how much muscle you have. That's a lot of factors, right? The most accurate way to figure out how many calories you should consume to lose weight is to find out your body fat percentage. Since it is pretty challenging to get an accurate reading, many people find they can lose weight successfully eating between 1,200 and 1,800 calories. I do not recommend 1,200 unless you are 5 feet 1 inch/155 cm or below.

Looking for a more accurate number? Your first step is calculating your BMR, basal metabolic rate. Your BMR is the minimum number of calories your body needs to function healthfully. My favorite is the Mifflin-St Jeor equation.

BMR = 10 x weight(kg) + 6.25 x height(cm) – 5 x age(y) + 5 (man)

BMR = 10 x weight(kg) + 6.25 x height(cm) – 5 x age(y) – 161 (woman)

To find your weight in kilograms, divide your weight in pounds by 2.2. To find your height in centimeters, multiply the number of inches by 2.54.

For a 25-year-old female, 5 feet 4 inches/162.5 cm and 140 pounds/63.6 kilograms, you would find your BMR using this equation: 10(63.6) + 6.25(162.5) – 125 –161 = BMR 1366. After you figure out your BMR, you need to determine your calorie requirements for weight loss.

If you are active and plan to follow my program, multiply that BMR number by 1.55. If you have a job that requires you to be on your feet all day, such as a nursing or waiting tables, then multiply it by 1.725. This is the total number of calories your body needs to maintain your weight. If you are just lightly exercising or on vacation, multiple that number by 1.375. If you are rehabbing an injury and are not exercising at all, multiple the number by 1.200 for your daily caloric needs to maintain your weight. If you eat less, you will lose weight. If you eat more, you will gain weight. Multiply this new number by .8 and .67 to get a range of calories you should be aiming to consume if you want to lose weight.

For the young woman in my example, who is following my program, this means she should be eating between 1,408 and 1,877 calories per day to lose 1 to 2 pounds/.5–1 kg a week. I suggest aiming for the middle of your range, and if you eat a little more or less, don't sweat it.

WHY SHOULD YOU COUNT YOUR CALORIES?

I do not regularly keep track of the number of calories I consume, but I do suggest it for those who are starting out on their weight-loss journey. It is very helpful, since many people underestimate the number they are consuming. I do use a food scale for portion control with nut butters, meats, fish and other difficult-to-measure items. I found out how many calories I should be consuming a few years ago for my body fat/muscle mass percentage. About once a month I track my calories for a day to make sure I'm staying accountable to myself.

HOW MANY MEALS A DAY SHOULD YOU EAT?

You should eat 3 meals a day and have 1 or 2 snacks, depending on your schedule. Allow at least 3 hours between meals. If you are going to go more than 4.5 hours without a meal, have a snack between meals. While I suggest eating a snack only if you are hungry, it is a good idea to plan ahead. Bring a smart snack in your purse if you know you'll be on the go. You may plan your snacks between breakfast and lunch, lunch and dinner; if you know you like a sweet treat at night, save one of your snacks for later in the evening. Just remember to have it at least 2 hours before going to bed to ensure that you get a restful sleep and wake up feeling fresh.

I am a firm believer in doing what works for you. Over the past few years, snacking has become a major component to many weight-loss programs, which cite its ability to stave of hunger and increase metabolism. However, snacking too much has taken away our ability to sense when we are actually hungry. Many people who have slowly and unknowingly gained weight and are starting this program should look closely at their snacking habits. Ask yourself if you are snacking even when you are not hungry or if your snacks contain over 300 calories. If so, it's time to rethink the "metabolism boosting" morsels that are sabotaging your efforts. We often snack on salty, processed foods and too often overindulge in such fare. It's important to give our stomachs time to digest after each meal. Constant snacking can disrupt digestion, leading to binging and causing rather than preventing cravings.

DO YOU NEED TO EAT BEFORE AND AFTER YOUR WORKOUTS?

The answer to the first part of this question will depend on the time of day, intensity and duration of your workout.

Eat before a workout if:

• You plan for an intense morning workout that will last longer than 30 minutes, such as spinning, sprint Intervals, boot camp

- A long workout at any time of day that will last longer than 75 minutes

- You're hungry!

Do not eat before a workout if:

- You're only doing an easy to moderate morning workout that will be completed within the first hour of waking up, such as yoga, barre class or a 30-minute jog

- You are not hungry.

- Unless you are training for a longer-distance race or intense workout, eat only when you are hungry before a workout. Working out on an empty stomach has shown to burn more fat when you do it within the first hour of waking up and it is not overly challenging. If you do eat, you will be able to work out harder, which is why it's important to do so if you are training for a race versus just trying to lose weight. Something like half a banana should suffice. I also love the Vega Pre-Workout Energy Drink. It's made with green tea and really gets me going. Black coffee or espresso can also energize your workout. Unless you have a heart condition, try having a cup 30 minutes before your workout for added energy for working harder and longer. I also love having my Energy Balls (page 175) before a workout, a slice of toast with peanut butter and jelly, or a green juice. You want your body to be able to digest whatever you eat quickly, which is why the simple sugars found in fruit are a great option.

- You should eat something after a workout if it's time for one of your meals or you worked out intensely for 60 minutes or more. You will get faster results if you do so. What you eat should have a ratio of 4–3 grams of carbs to 1 gram of protein. Don't overanalyze this; just make sure your recovery includes protein and carbs. These calories should be included in what you are aiming to eat for the day. Just because you work out does not mean you get to eat the number of calories you just burned in addition to your previous calculation. Plan your workout so that you will be eating one of your meals or snacks within an hour of finishing up. Keep snacks at between 150 and 200 calories and meals at between 300 and 400 calories.

- If you work out at a gym that is not close to home or head to work afterward, bring a packet of protein powder to mix in your water bottle after you finish, as you shower and get dressed. You can also bring a protein bar or an Energy Ball. This is important because refueling after a workout helps your muscles recover and rebuild. See my snack suggestions below for ideas.

TIME TO DO SOME HOMEWORK
MEAL PREP TIPS

1. Plan your weekday meals ahead of time.

2. Make multiple servings of each dish so that you have leftovers for lunch or dinner later in the week.

3. Give each week a theme so fresh ingredients are not wasted. For example, plan a week of Mexican dinners including a taco salad, a quesadilla, tacos and so on.

At the end of this chapter I've included a shopping list of all the items that I typically buy. I do not buy the entire list each time I visit a grocery store. It depends on what I have already at home, what I've planned and how many meals I am going to be eating out. You will probably need to buy many of the items only once every two weeks or less frequently if they are nonperishable, like quinoa.

DO I RECOMMEND ANY SPECIFIC DIET?

Some days I eat vegan, others I eat gluten-free or paleo. This is not intentional; I don't believe in putting a label on my diet, but by nature it is one that is plant-based. If you have an allergy or dietary preference, there are substitutions provided below . Aim to eat most of your complex carbohydrates at breakfast and lunch. Carbs are not the enemy! Do not be afraid of any macro-nutrient. Fat and carbs have been attacked recently, but your body needs fat to burn fat, and it needs carbs to energize your workouts so you can get skinny again. Aim for 30–40% of calories to come from protein, 30–40% from carbohydrates and 20–30% from fat.

After hearing some not-so-pleasant information on how animals are raised in factory farms, if I am eating out at a restaurant and have no idea where the meat came from, I will usually choose shellfish or vegetarian entrées.

When I'm at the grocery store, these are the rules I follow: avoid fish that is farm-raised; choose beef that is grass-fed, hormone-free and organic if it is available; select poultry that is free-range and organic; and always buy organic soy products.

Eat lean protein simply prepared with spices and natural condiments that add flavor such as Dijon mustard, salsa or vinegar. These condiments and spices boost flavor and add virtually no calories to your meals. I've included my favorite ones, which I use regularly in my recipes, in my shopping list.

Your dinner does not have to come from a recipe. None of your meals does. You probably do not need directions to grill salmon and steam broccoli, but having condiments on hand can make them crave-worthy favorites.

THE MEALS

Every diet book out there has a crazy list of recipes that require too many ingredients. You make the recipe once and then the other half of that parsley bunch goes bad before you can buy the rest of the ingredients to make it again. My meal ideas are so simple that you will always have the ingredients on hand and be able to eat clean.

BREAKFAST

First thing when you wake up, have a cup of warm-to-hot water with freshly squeezed lemon juice to wake up your body and get things moving. Wait about 30 minutes before eating anything unless you are planning to work out hard for longer than 30 minutes. Waiting allows the lemon juice

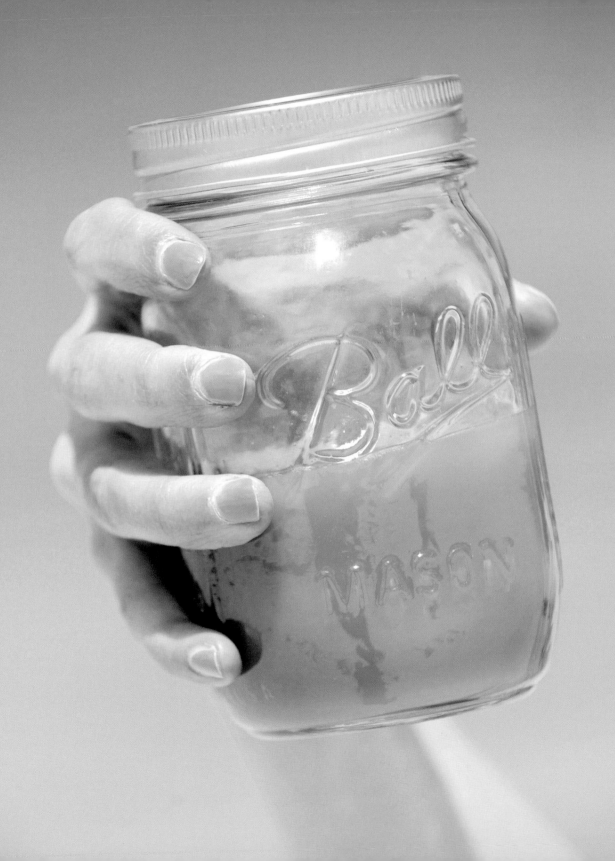

to stimulate the gastrointestinal tract on an empty stomach, which helps improve digestion and encourages your bowels to eliminate toxins and waste. You should eat breakfast within an hour of waking up. This allows you time to get in a quick workout using any stored energy that you didn't use the day before: you can burn some of your fat stores before using muscle for energy.

These breakfasts are between 150 and 300 calories and will keep you feeling full until lunchtime!

- 2 slices of Ezekiel bread with 1 tablespoon/16 grams of natural peanut butter (no sugar or oils added)

- Oatmeal with fixings. I like to add flax or chia seeds, berries, nuts, cottage cheese, coconut flakes or protein powder

- Low-fat Greek yogurt with fruit and nuts

- Tropical Green Smoothie (page 168)

- Big bowl of fruit

- 1 egg plus 2 egg whites (cooked however you like) on a slice of Ezekiel bread with avocado and sprouts

- Smoothie. See pages 168-169 for suggestions

- Protein Pancake (page 167)

- On-the-Go Protein Muffins (page 170)

- Kale and Quinoa Frittata (page 171)

If you are eating breakfast on the go, here are a few suggestions that will help you stick to your plan.

- Diner: Egg-white omelet with veggies and fruit

- Starbucks: Oatmeal or Spinach-and-Feta Wrap

- Dunkin' Donuts: Egg-White Flatbread

- Bagel Shop: Scooped-out whole-wheat bagel with low-fat cream cheese, hummus or tofu spread

LUNCH AT HOME

This is the most frequent meal eaten outside the home. Try to pack a lunch for the day or look at online menus so that you know what you will be eating. I prefer to have at least one big salad a day, and that usually ends up being my lunch. Aim to consume at least 2 cups/70–150 g (depending on the vegetable) of nonstarchy vegetables. Add lean protein that is about the size of a deck of cards. Grilled chicken, tofu, tuna, turkey, tempeh, egg whites or beans are good sources. Add about 2 teaspoons/10 ml of olive oil, a quarter of an avocado or 1 tablespoon/15 g of nuts, such as walnuts. Make your own salad dressing (see my easy recipe, page 174) or buy a low-fat alternative.

Avoid fat-free dressings, as they are filled with sugar. You can also try just using lemon juice or hummus mixed with mashed avocado and you will not miss a thing. A large salad can take a while to prepare in the morning, so here are my favorite quick-fix lunches to take to school or work. You'll find some of the recipes in the next section.

• Leafy greens with hummus, tabouli, and water-packed tuna

• Chicken Salad or No-Chop Healthy Tuna Salad (page 172) on top of greens or Ezekiel bread

• Low-Carb Turkey Wrap (page 171)

• Summer Quinoa Salad (page 173)

• Brown rice sushi or sashimi (4–6 pieces) with miso soup and seaweed salad

• Salsa Chicken Quesadilla (page 178), with grape tomatoes

LUNCH OUT

• Panera Bread Hidden Menu Power Chicken Hummus Bowl

• Au Bon Pain Vegetarian Deluxe Salad with Light Lemon Shallot or Balsamic Vinaigrette Dressing

• Così Hummus & Veggies Sandwich

• Pret A Manger Albacore Tuna Niçoise Salad with Skinny Vinaigrette

• Subway 6-inch Turkey Breast on 9-Grain Wheat with avocado (no cheese)

• Starbucks Zesty Chicken and Black Bean Salad Bowl

SNACK TIME

Snacks can make or break a diet. If you are starving, eat something! Too often, though, we eat a snack based on the clock and not how we feel. Here are my favorite go-to snack options for natural energy during the day. These are all between 150 and 250 calories.

• Celery or apple with 2 tablespoons/32 grams peanut butter

• Carrots with 4 tablespoons/60 grams hummus

• One-quarter cup/60 grams dried edamame with half a banana

• 15 almonds with an orange

• 10 walnut halves

• 2 hard-boiled eggs

• Protein shake or smoothie made with water or unsweetened almond milk

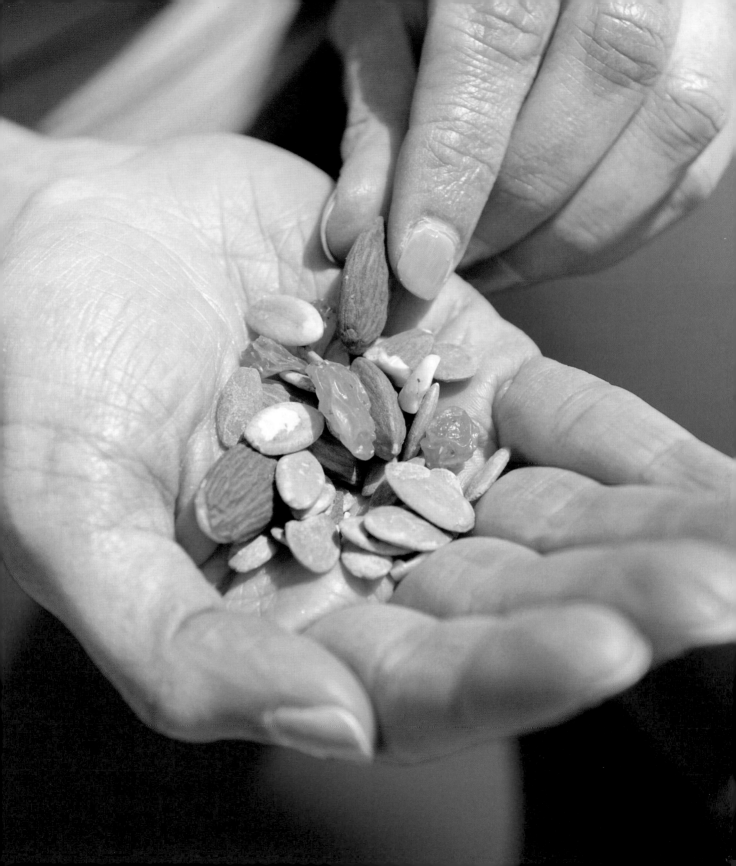

- Tropical Green Smoothie (page 168)

- Wrap made with 3 thin slices of turkey and a dollop of hummus in the middle

- Cottage cheese or Greek yogurt with berries (if not eaten for breakfast)

- Energy or protein bar

- Portion-controlled trail mix (around 200–250 calories)

- 1 piece Mini Babybel Cheese Light Original with two Clementines

- 2 Energy Balls (page 175)

- Fruit and Nut Fit Granola Bars (page 176)

DINNER

Eat dinner at least 2 hours before going to bed and avoid starches while trying to drop down to your feel-skinny weight. Eating too close to bedtime can cause indigestion and may interfere with a restful night's sleep. Waking up tired may lead to a day of overeating; you are far more likely to wake up feeling energized and fresh when you stop eating and give your body sufficient time to digest before lying down. Have 4 ounces/115 grams of a lean protein (the size of your palm) and 2 cups/70–150 g) of green veggies. Having half a sweet potato or half a cup/90 grams of cooked quinoa, lentils or beans is fine as well. If you love your starchy carbs, eat them at breakfast or lunch.

Any green vegetable is a great choice to eat at dinner, such as broccoli, asparagus, Brussels sprouts or kale. Steam, roast or sauté with a little extra virgin olive oil. Add salt and pepper to taste. Stock your freezer with frozen broccoli, asparagus and kale for busy weeks when you don't have time to go grocery shopping. I also usually have fish and chicken in the freezer, too.

The best protein options are shrimp, flaky white fish, chicken, lean beef, pork, tofu, tempeh, beans and seitan.

Here are my favorite dinner recipes and ideas:

- Salsa Chicken Mexican Salad (page 177)

- Buffalo Turkey Meatloaf (page 182) with a veggie

- Baked wild salmon with tzatziki sauce and a side of roasted beets

- Roasted or sautéed chicken breast topped with store-bought jarred bruschetta topping

- Shrimp or chicken and vegetable teriyaki stir-fry

- Spaghetti squash or Eggplant Pasta (page 179) with low-sugar tomato sauce and meatless meatballs

- Veggie burger or chicken patty with Sweet Potato Fries (page 180) and broccoli

- Cheesy Butternut Squash Quinoa (page 181)

Tip for college students: If you are going out for the night and know you have a tendency to crave pizza once you get home, be prepared. Keep a low-sugar pasta sauce in stock. Then, when you get home from your night out, make your own mini-pizza with English muffins (preferably Ezekiel), the pasta sauce and a Mini Babybel cheese round on top. Place in the microwave (or the oven, if you are sober) and voilà! You have a delicious, healthy alternative to feed your late-night craving.

If you are eating dinner out at a restaurant, see my guide in chapter 6, "Time to Be Social."

SWEET ENDINGS

I am a dessert girl. It's hard for me to say no to homemade baked goods. However, when I'm at home, it's easy to indulge a craving for sweets for a fraction of the calories with nutritious foods. Here are my favorite go-to sweet treats that do not contain empty calories.

- Instant Pumpkin Pie Mousse (page 184)

- Chia Pudding (page 183)

- High-Protein Frozen Banana Soft-Serve (page 185)

- 1 tablespoon/16 grams peanut butter and 1 tablespoon/15 grams protein powder mixed to make fudge

INGREDIENT SUBSTITUTES

Below are a few ingredients that I use pretty frequently in my recipes. If you do not have them, do not like them, or are allergic to them, substitutions as well as what to look for when buying them are offered.

Unsweetened almond milk: You can use unsweetened coconut milk, organic soy milk, hemp milk, 2% or 1% dairy milk. If the recipe calls for unsweetened vanilla and you're using regular, add a dash of vanilla extract. Do not buy the sweetened versions, as they contain unnecessary added sugar.

Eggs or egg whites: I buy organic eggs all the time. It's worth the money if you can afford it. If you are a vegan, try using a flax egg. Mix 1 tablespoon/20 g of flaxseed meal with 3 tablespoons/15 ml of warm water. Whisk together for a minute and let sit for 5 minutes. Warning: this substitution may not work for all recipes, such as the Kale and Quniona Frittata, but it works great for the Post Workout On-the-go Protein Muffin.

Peanut butter: Buy unsalted, unsweetened and sans extra oil. Nut butters are naturally sweet on their own. For most of the recipes you can swap in any nut butter you like, including but not limited to sunflower butter, cashew butter, almond butter and coconut butter. The ingredients label should have only one ingredient.

Protein powder: If you do not want to use protein powder, feel free to use Greek yogurt in smoothies or oat flour, almond meal or coconut flour in the baking recipes. You may have to add a little extra sweetener for the best taste. If you are unfamiliar with protein powder, it's a very versatile ingredient that boosts protein content and can be used in place of flour or even sugar sometimes. Amazing in smoothies, it can be used in my breakfast and snack recipes to increase the protein in an otherwise carb-heavy dish. My current favorite brands are Perfect Fit, Vega, Jay Robb and Designer Whey.

Oat flour: You can buy this in a store premade, or you can make it yourself if you have a blender or food processor. Just pour a cup of old-fashioned or quick-cooking oats into a blender or food processor and process until they have a flourlike consistency. You can of course use regular flour, whole wheat flour, almond meal, peanut flour, gluten-free flour, amaranth flour or any other flour, for that matter.

Stevia drops: You can buy stevia drops at Whole Foods or online. I use NuNaturals and love them. They last forever! I use them to sweeten my Greek yogurt, tea, homemade desserts and more. If you cannot find them, you can use half of one granulated stevia packet in place of 2–4 drops. A full packet can be used in place of 6–8 drops. Other alternatives are honey, agave nectar and regular sugar.

RECIPES

PROTEIN PANCAKE (SERVES 1)

This is one of my go-to breakfasts after a morning workout. If you do not like bananas, you can substitute 3 tablespoons/44 g of cooked oatmeal, applesauce or canned pumpkin. Leave the skin on when you cut the banana and save the other half in the refrigerator, or take the peel off and freeze it for a smoothie. It's also great as a dessert if you are craving something sweet after dinner.

½ medium banana

1 egg white (or substitute 3 tbsp/45 ml liquid egg whites)

1 scoop vanilla protein powder

2 tbsp/30 ml unsweetened vanilla almond milk (or substitute coconut milk)

optional additions: 1 tsp/2.5 g cinnamon, 1 tbsp/7 g flaxseed meal, 1 tbsp/10 g chia seeds, 1 tbsp / 10 g frozen blueberries, 1 tsp/5 g nut butter

Preheat a skillet on medium heat. Combine all ingredients except milk in a deep bowl and blend well with a large fork, whisk, or use immersion blender for a smooth consistency. If batter is too dry or you want thinner pancakes, add the milk. Depending on the brand of your protein powder, you may need less or more almond milk for your preferred consistency. If you're using the cinnamon, flaxseed meal, or chia seeds, add them now. Spray pan with coconut oil or other nonstick spray and pour half the batter into the skillet. Sprinkle blueberries on top if desired. Once edges look firm (about 2–3 minutes), flip and finish cooking for another minute. Repeat with the remaining batter. You may make one large pancake, but it may be hard to flip.

TIP: If you spray the coconut or canola oil onto the skillet and it turns brown, the pan is too hot and the pancake will taste burnt. Wash off the oil and warm it up again.

Nutrition per serving (does not include optional additions): 145 Calories, 16g Carbs, 0g Fat, 20 g Protein, 4g Fiber, 7g Sugar

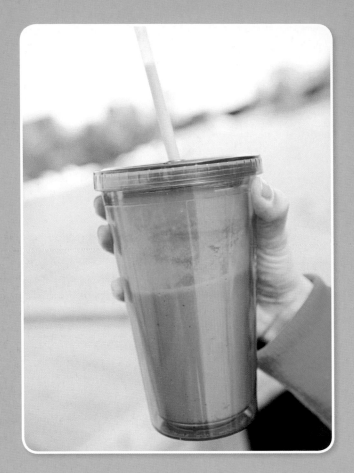

TROPICAL GREEN SMOOTHIE (SERVES 1)

This is a gluten-free, vegan meal made with fresh fruits and veggies. You will be amazed that you cannot taste the spinach. This is one of my favorite go-to meals for breakfast, lunch or after a workout. It's sweet, filling and full of nutrients that your body will use to burn fat and help you look long and lean.

1 scoop protein powder, vanilla or fruit flavored

¼ cup/40 g frozen mango or pineapple

1 cup/30 g fresh spinach

½ medium frozen banana

1 cup/240 ml unsweetened vanilla almond milk

4 ice cubes

Combine ingredients in a blender. You may add avocado, flaxseeds or chia seeds if you want extra fiber and heart-healthy fats. Add 1-3 tablespoons/15–45 ml of water if you want a thinner smoothie. Blend well until it's a smooth consistency.

Nutrition per serving: 175 Calories, 22g Carbs, 3g Fat, 18g Protein, 5.5g Fiber 11g Sugar

PEANUT BUTTER AND JELLY TIME SMOOTHIE (SERVES 1)

This smoothie does not have protein powder but is still high in protein from the Greek yogurt and peanut butter. It reminds me of my favorite sandwich growing up.

1 cup/152 g frozen or fresh strawberries

1 tbsp/16 g peanut butter

1 tbsp/10 g chia seeds

1 cup/227 g nonfat plain Greek yogurt

1 cup/240 ml almond milk

4 ice cubes

Combine all ingredients in a blender. Blend well until smooth.

Nutrition per serving: 256 Calories, 14g Carbs, 16g Fat, 14g Protein, 10g Fiber, 6g Sugar

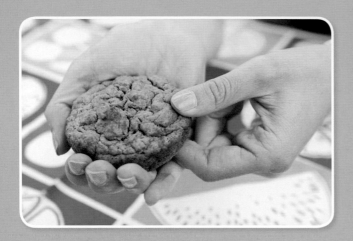

POST-WORKOUT ON-THE-GO PROTEIN MUFFINS (SERVES 4–6)

These are great for having after a morning workout on your way to class or work. I like to make them to have for breakfast when I travel. They have a few more ingredients than the rest of my recipes, but they are worth it. You can omit the flaxseed, cinnamon and blueberries if you want but the taste won't be as amazing!

1½ medium bananas

3 egg whites (or ½ cup/120 ml liquid egg whites)

½ cup/177 g cooked steel-cut or old-fashioned oats

½ cup/120 g protein powder

3 tbsp/21 g flaxseed meal

1 tbsp/7 g cinnamon

1 tsp/3.7 g baking soda

Dash of salt

¼ cup/40 g frozen blueberries

Preheat oven to 350°F/177°C. Combine banana, egg whites and oatmeal. Blend with a whisk, immersion blender or food processor until the mixture becomes smooth. In a separate bowl, combine protein powder, flaxseed meal, cinnamon, baking soda and salt. Mix with a fork or spoon thoroughly. Combine the wet and dry ingredients. Grease large muffin tin with coconut or canola oil or other nonstick oil spray. Pour batter evenly into muffin cups. Add frozen blueberries on top of the batter. Bake for 25 minutes. Check after 20 minutes; depending on your oven, it may take up to 35 minutes for the tops of the muffins to become golden.

Nutrition per serving: 167 Calories, 22g Carbs, 3g Fat, 14g Protein, 6g Fiber, 7g Sugar

KALE AND QUINOA FRITTATA (SERVES 6)

This recipe is much lighter than your average quiche. By eliminating the crust and using almond milk and Laughing Cow cheese, there are less calories without sacrificing taste. Make this dish on Sunday night for a ready-to-go breakfast all week. Pair with a salad for a filling lunch or dinner, too!

¼ cup/42.5 g uncooked quinoa

½ cup/120 ml water

1 small onion, diced
½ tsp/2.5 ml extra virgin olive oil

1 cup/67 g kale, stems removed and thinly sliced
1 garlic clove, chopped

2 eggs

4 egg whites

1 cup/240 ml unsweetened almond milk

4 wedges Laughing Cow Light

1 tsp/5 g salt

½ tsp/1q pepper

Dash of cayenne

Rinse quinoa and add to a small pot with the water. Cover. Bring to a boil and then turn heat down to simmer for 15 minutes or until quinoa is plump and ready. Preheat oven to 400°F/204°C. While quinoa is cooking, sauté onion in oil until softened. Add garlic and kale to sautéed onions. Cook for an additional 3–5 minutes, or until kale is wilted. Spray a pie plate or 3 large muffin cups with extra virgin olive oil. Evenly divide quinoa and place in the bottom of the pie plate or each muffin cup. Combine the eggs, egg whites, milk, cheese wedges, salt, pepper and cayenne. Blend well with a whisk or blender until cheese is broken up and the mixture is consistent throughout. Add the sautéed veggies to the egg mixture and stir. Pour mixture into pie plate or evenly in muffin cups. Bake in the center of your oven at 400°F/204°C for 15 minutes, then turn down to 350°F/177°C for an additional 25 minutes. You may need less time if making this recipe in a muffin tin. (Note: one muffin serves 2.)

Nutrition per serving: 115 Calories, 4g Fat, 11g Carbs, 8g Protein, 2g Fiber, 4g Sugar

NO-CHOP HEALTHY TUNA SALAD (SERVES 1)

I love tuna salad, but I hate cutting up celery and onion. I know I sound lazy, but in the morning when I'm on my way out the door, I want something simple when I'm choosing what to take with me for lunch. I created a delicious and simple tuna recipe that involves no chopping so that I can still have a sandwich for lunch when I am running late.

1 (2.5 oz) can tuna, unsalted and water-packed

1 tbsp/15 g hummus

1 tsp/5.2 g Dijon mustard

salt and pepper to taste

Mix tuna, hummus and mustard well until tuna is no longer clumpy and season to taste. I love to put this between two slices of Ezekiel bread with a side of grape tomatoes for a quick lunch.

Nutrition per serving (not including bread in serving suggestion): 130 Calories, 3g Carbs, 7g Fat, 15g Protein, 1g Fiber, 0g Sugar

GREEN GODDESS CHICKEN SALAD (SERVES 2)

This is an easy way to make your chicken breasts go a long way. The Greek yogurt adds extra protein and the avocado contributes heart-healthy fats and flavor. Serve this on top of lettuce greens or in a high-fiber wrap.

1 (6-7 oz/170-198 g) skinless, boneless chicken breast

3 tbsp/43 g nonfat plain Greek yogurt

½ avocado, chopped (about 2 oz./60 g)

1 tbsp/2.5 g parsley, chopped

1 tsp/5 ml lemon juice (optional)

Salt and pepper to taste

Bake chicken breast and let cool. Chop chicken into small cubes and combine in a bowl with the Greek yogurt, avocado, parsley and lemon juice if using. Add salt and pepper to taste. Don't let the parsley go to waste—make the Summer Quinoa Salad the same week.

Nutrition per serving: 146 Calories, 5g Carbs, 9g Fat, 20g Protein, 3g Fiber, 1g Sugar

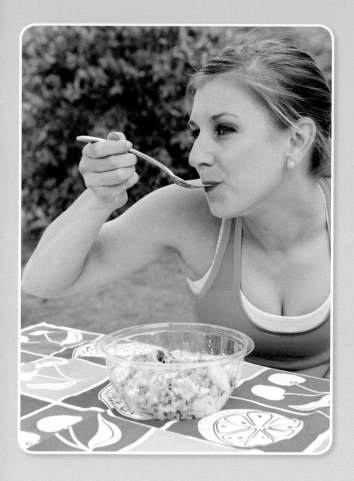

SUMMER QUINOA SALAD (SERVES 4)

This is great for a side dish or one-bowl meal.

½ cup/85 g quinoa, uncooked

1 yellow or orange bell pepper, chopped

½ cup/75 g red onion, chopped

¼ cup/10 g parsley, stems removed and finely chopped

1 tbsp/15 ml lemon juice

½ tsp/2.6 g Dijon mustard

2 tbsp/30 ml extra virgin olive oil

1 tbsp/8.6 g raw pepitas or other nut or seed (optional)

¼ avocado, sliced (optional)

Cook quinoa according to package and set aside in a large bowl. Finely chop bell pepper and red onion. Add bell pepper, onion and parsley to quinoa. Blend well. Combine the lemon juice, Dijon mustard and olive oil. Drizzle over quinoa mixture. Toss until well blended. Refrigerate until ready to serve. Eat this as is for a side dish or add pepitas and avocado and 3 ounces/84 g of protein for a delicious meal. I like tofu, shrimp or grilled chicken in this salad.

Nutrition per serving: 110 Calories, 10g Carbs, 7g Fat, 2g Protein, 1.5g Fiber, 1g Sugar

LO-CARB TURKEY WRAP (SERVES 1)

This is my go-to sandwich in the summer. It's quick to make in the morning and does not get soggy. Feel free to add avocado or red onion if you're not in a rush.

1 high-fiber whole-wheat wrap, 60–70 calories

1 thin slice light Swiss cheese (or use a spreadable light wedge such as Laughing Cow)

1 tbsp/16 g Dijon or honey mustard

2 oz/56 g deli sliced turkey breast (3–4 slices)

¼ cup/8 g sprouts, thoroughly washed and dried

Lay the wrap flat on the countertop. Place the Swiss cheese directly in the center. Spread the mustard, more or less if you like, on the cheese. Add the turkey and top with the sprouts. Roll up the wrap and you're ready to rock.

Nutrition per serving: 178 Calories, 13 g Carbs, 6g Fat, 22g Protein, 7g Fiber, 2g Sugar

SIMPLE HOMEMADE SALAD DRESSING (SERVES 1)

When I run out of salad dressing or feel guilty about being lazy and buying it so often, I make this simple, low-calorie hummus dressing. Vinegar is very cheap, but making homemade dressing taste good without a ton of oil is a challenge. I'd rather get my healthy fats from nuts or an avocado, so I've settled on this quick fix. It goes well on many salads.

2 tbsp/30 g hummus

1 tsp/5 g Dijon mustard

2 tbsp/30 ml balsamic vinegar

Combine all 3 ingredients in a bowl and blend well. This is delicious over a salad of spring-mix lettuces, left-over sweet potato fries (page 180), sun-dried tomatoes, sliced or chopped cucumber, sliced red onion, and water-packed tuna.

Nutrition per serving: 181 Calories, 19 g Carbs, 10g Fat, 4g Protein, 4g Fiber, 2g Sugar

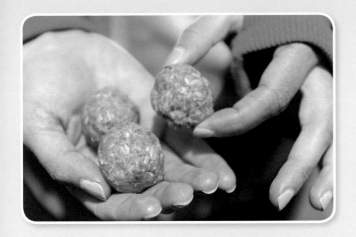

ENERGY BALLS (MAKES 12 BALLS/SERVINGS)

This recipe is decadent. It's rich and sweet and tastes like a truffle. Best of all, it's vegan, and you don't have to bake it! These are perfect as pre-workout energizers. If you have an early-morning session, just pop one in your mouth and you'll be ready to crush it. They are also easy to pack, as they do not take up much space. I prefer to keep them refrigerated, but a few hours in your purse won't hurt them, and they're perfect for an afternoon snack to fuel an after-workout run.

4 tbsp/64 g peanut butter

½ cup/120 g protein powder, vanilla or chocolate

¼ cup/45 g oat flour or ½ cup/45 g old-fashioned oats

1 tsp/5 ml vanilla extract

4 tsp/20 ml honey

½ tsp/2.5 g sea salt (I like Himalayan)

¼ cup/60 ml unsweetened almond milk or water (you may need more depending on protein powder)

If you do not have oat flour, you can grind the oats in a food processor to make oat flour. Combine all the ingredients except for the almond milk in a bowl and mix together with a spoon. If you need to, add almond milk or water a teaspoon at a time until mixture is no longer crumbling. Scoop out about 1 tablespoon of batter and roll into a tight ball. Repeat with the remaining batter. You can eat these right away or place in an air-tight container in the refrigerator to harden up a bit.

This is a basic recipe—you can add chocolate chips, coconut flakes, chia seeds or flax, if you like, for your own spin.

Nutrition per serving: 81 calories, 8 g Carbs, 4g Fat, 5g Protein, 1g Fiber, 4g Sugar

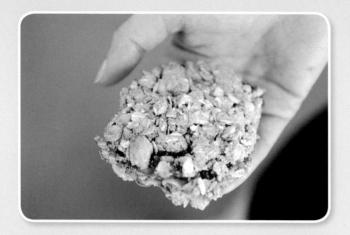

FRUIT AND NUT FIT GRANOLA BARS (MAKES 12 BARS)

These are great for a post-workout snack on the go. This is an excellent base for any granola bar.

1 medium banana

2 tbsp/42.6 g honey

½ cup/120 ml unsweetened almond milk

1½/120 g cups old-fashioned or quick-cooking oats

¼ cup/60 g vanilla protein powder

½ cup/45 g oat flour

½ cup/75 g sliced almonds

½ cup/75 g raisins or other chopped dried fruits

Preheat oven to 350°F/177°C. In a large bowl combine banana, honey and almond milk. Blend well with a whisk, immersion blender or food processor. Combine oats, protein powder, oat flour, almonds and raisins. Combine the wet and dry ingredients. Pour the mixture into a greased 9×9-inch/23×23-cm pan and press it down firmly and evenly. Bake for 20 minutes or until it is of desired crispiness. Let cool and cut into 12 squares or bars . I like to cut these into single-serving portions and put each portion in a plastic baggie to go.

Nutrition per serving: 125 Calories, 4g Fat, 20 Carbs, 3g Fiber, 7g Sugar, 6g Protein

SALSA CHICKEN (SERVES 6)

If you have a slow-cooker, this meal is a must! Its a staple in my house because of its affordability, versatility and flavor. I use it for salads, burrito bowls on top of quinoa, in lettuce wraps with avocado and in quesadillas. You can also use it to make homemade chili.

2 lbs/896 g boneless, skinless chicken breasts

1 jar (16 oz/420 g) salsa (use your favorite, fruity or spicy, doesn't matter, or make your own)

Pour out a little bit of salsa on the bottom of the slow cooker to cover the surface. Next, place the chicken breasts on top so that they are not overlapping. Cover with the rest of the salsa in the jar. Place the lid on top and set slow cooker to low. After about 6 hours on low, remove the chicken from the cooker and pull the chicken breasts apart with two forks. This should be easy to do—the chicken should just fall apart. If you try to do this too early, you will have to use some force and the chicken may end up tasting kind of dry. Return chicken to slow cooker and cook for another hour. Remove chicken and salsa from the slow cooker and turn off the cooker. If you cook this on high, check the chicken after 3 hours and pull apart if it's ready. If you are home during the cooking process, you can rotate the chicken in the pot with a pair of tongs, but do not pierce the breasts until the final stage.

Nutrition per serving: 135 Calories, 1g Fat, 3g Carbs, 24g Protein, 0g Fiber, 1g Sugar

SALSA CHICKEN MEXICAN SALAD (SERVES 1)

If you are looking for a filling dinner, I highly recommend this large salad. For extra crunch I top it with a few tortilla chips. If you have bell peppers or onions on hand, you can include them. You can also omit the Greek yogurt or ranch dressing if you do not eat dairy.

2 cups/94 g romaine lettuce

½ cup/115 g Salsa Chicken

1 tbsp/10 g sliced jalapeño peppers (or to taste)

¼ avocado

3 tbsp/45 g fresh salsa

1 tbsp/28 g plain Greek yogurt or yogurt-based ranch dressing

Wash and chop the lettuce and place in a bowl. Top with salsa chicken, jalapeños and avocado. Mix fresh salsa with Greek yogurt or ranch dressing for a creamy dressing and drizzle on top. If you have tortilla chips, add a few on top for crunch.

Nutrition per serving: 232 Calories, 11g Fat, 13g Carbs, 27g Protein, 4g Fiber, 6g Sugar

SALSA CHICKEN QUESADILLA (SERVES 1)

Looking for a quick meal? This quesadilla is easy, cheap and delicious. Have it for lunch on the weekend to kill a comfort food craving for under 200 calories.

¼ cup/57 g Salsa Chicken

1 wedge Laughing Cow Light Queso Fresco and Chipotle

1 high-fiber whole-grain tortilla

Preheat a pan on medium heat. Smear cheese on one side of the tortilla. Spread chicken over cheese on one half of the tortilla and fold the tortilla to look like a half moon. Spray the heated pan with olive and place the tortilla in the pan. Cook for 3 minutes and flip. Cook the opposite side until the tortilla is brown and crispy. Feel free to add extra veggies in the quesadilla. Serve with salsa and avocado.

Nutrition per serving: 205 Calories, 10g Carbs, 7g Fat, 26g Protein, 12g Fiber, 3g Sugar

EGGPLANT PASTA (SERVES 1)

I love tomato sauce and veggie-rich pasta dishes but I find boxed pasta to be boring and flavorless. Using veggies such as zucchini or eggplant, is a great way to enjoy typical Italian pasta dishes without the empty calories. Use this recipe in place of pasta for some of your family favorite meals.

1 medium eggplant

Salt

½ tbsp/7.5 ml olive oil

1 cup/236 g homemade or low-sugar pasta sauce (Whole Foods Roasted Vegetable is my favorite)

Peel eggplant, leaving about 2 inches/5 cm of skin at both ends. Thinly slice the long way so that pieces are about ¼ inch/.64 cm thick. Lay eggplant pieces flat on a cooling rack or paper towels. Sprinkle generously with salt. After 15–20 minutes, rinse the eggplant well, brushing off the salt. Squeeze out the excess moisture by pressing down hard on the slices and pat the eggplant dry. Preheat a large skillet to medium with the oil. Line up the eggplant pieces and cut into very thin strips that look like fettuccini. Add strips of eggplant to the skillet and sauté on medium-low for about 8–10 minutes, or until eggplant is completely wilted. Add tomato sauce and cook for another minute or until sauce is hot.

Make this a complete meal by adding veggie meatballs, lean ground beef or shrimp. It can also be used as a side to an Italian-inspired main course.

Nutrition per serving: 150 Calories, 26g Carbs, 6g Fat, 5g Protein, 15.6g Fiber, 11 g Sugar

SWEET POTATO FRIES (SERVES 2)

This is a go-to recipe of mine. It's also a little family gem. The secrets to great sweet potato fries are cutting them thin enough that they get crispy, even though they're not fried, and using allspice. Allspice is not something you will use often, but if you make these as often as I do (about once a week), it will be well worth the money. This is an excellent side dish to accompany a simple baked protein like fish or chicken with tzatziki, teriyaki or barbeque sauce.

1 medium sweet potato

¼ tsp/.5 g allspice

Salt and pepper to taste

1 tsp/5 ml olive oil

Preheat your oven to 400°F/204°C. Scrub sweet potato under cold running water to remove any excess dirt. Cut in half the long way. With the flat surface facing down, begin to carefully slice sweet potato into thin strips. You may also cut it into small home fry–like rectangular shapes, which will be easier to chop and cook faster. In a large bowl toss together sweet potato strips, the allspice, salt and pepper. Try to coat each piece evenly but don't stress about it too much. Add the olive oil and toss well. Line a large cookie sheet with sweet potato strips in a single layer. Bake for 15 minutes. Turn the fries over and bake for another 10 minutes, or until they have reached the desired crispiness. Save the leftovers to add to a salad or save for dinner later in the week.

Nutrition per serving: 102 Calories, 19g Carbs, 3g Fat, 2g Protein, 3g Fiber, 8g Sugar

CHEESY BUTTERNUT SQUASH QUINOA (SERVES 2)

This is a great comfort-food dinner without the guilt. You can avoid having to cut up the butternut squash by purchasing it precut. In the fall squash is in season in New England, so I always try to buy mine at a local farmers' market.

3 cups/420 g butternut squash, peeled and cubed

Salt and pepper to taste

¼ tsp/.5 g allspice (optional)

¼ cup/42.5 g quinoa

1 cup/240 ml low-sodium chicken broth or water

½ cup/76 g onion, chopped

2 wedges Laughing Cow Light Swiss

1 cup/30 g baby spinach

1 tsp/1 g dried sage, rosemary or thyme (optional)

Handful of walnuts (optional)

Preheat oven to 400°F/204°C. Place squash on a cookie sheet sprayed with olive oil. Sprinkle potatoes with salt, pepper and the allspice (if using). Roast in oven for 25-30 minutes. Then set aside and preheat a medium-size pot on medium and spray with olive oil. Add onion and sauté for 5 minutes on medium-low, or until it is soft. Rinse quinoa under cold running water. Add quinoa and chicken broth or water to pot. Cover and bring to a boil. Reduce heat and simmer for 15 minutes. Once broth has been absorbed, reduce heat as low as possible. Add cheese wedges and blend well. Add baby spinach and dried herb, if using. Add the roasted, seasoned squash to the pot, mashing some but not all the cubes. If the pot is too small, transfer the mixture to a large bowl. Mix thoroughly, but be sure to leave some of the squash unmashed. Sprinkle with walnuts.

Nutrition per serving: 267 Calories, 54g Carbs, 4g Fat, 10g Protein, 3g Fiber, 11g Sugar

BUFFALO TURKEY MEATLOAF (SERVES 4-6)

This recipe is so simple to make yet is bursting with flavor. It's also pretty cheap. Make it at the beginning of the week and enjoy the leftovers for lunch and dinner. Have it with a side dish of steamed broccoli or put it on top of a salad. Have 1 to 1½ muffin cups as a serving, depending on your hunger level.

½ cup/50 g chopped celery

½ cup/75 g chopped onion

1 egg

½ cup/40 g old-fashioned oats

¼ cup/59 ml hot sauce, such as Cholula or Frank's

½ tbsp/4 g garlic powder

1-1.25 lbs/452-565 g ground turkey (or chicken)

Preheat oven to 350°F/177°C. Combine all ingredients except turkey in a bowl and mix together. (You can often buy celery and onion already diced and sold together. This saves a step and sometimes it's worth it for me.) Add the turkey. Make sure the consistency is the same throughout. Evenly distribute mixture in 6 muffin cups. Bake for 25 minutes.

Nutrition per serving: 178 Calories, 7g Carbs, 8g Fat, 21g Protein, 1g Fiber, 1g Sugar

CHIA PUDDING (SERVES 1)

Eating nutritious desserts is one of the ways that I was able to successfully lose weight. Having safe and healthy options prevents you from grabbing something that will sabotage your efforts. This chia recipe is one you have to make to see for yourself.

2 tbsp/20 g chia seeds

2-3 drops stevia

6 tbsp/90 ml unsweetened almond milk

Handful of nuts or coconut flakes (optional)

In an airtight container, combine all the ingredients and put the lid on top. Refrigerate for at least 15 minutes, ideally an hour. The longer you wait, the more the chia seeds will expand and gel. This is best when it's cold. Eat it on its own as a pudding or add the mixture to some canned pumpkin or peanut butter for a sweet ending to the day. If you do not have stevia drops, you can use one of the alternatives listed under "Ingredient Substitutes" (page 165-166).

Nutrition per serving (without optional ingredients): 170 Calories, 3g Carbs, 13g Fat, 7g Protein, 13g Fiber, 0g Sugar

INSTANT PUMPKIN PIE MOUSSE (SERVES 1)

My body craves this dessert in the fall. I will have a protein and green veggie for dinner. But instead of having a sweet potato with my meal, I'll use a little canned pumpkin in this instant dessert that I can make for one.

½ cup/123 g canned pumpkin

2 tsp/10 g nut butter, such as peanut, cashew or almond

2 tbsp/30 ml almond milk

Dash cinnamon

2–3 drops stevia

In a small bowl, combine all the ingredients and stir together until the mixture is smooth. If you do not have stevia drops, you can use one of the alternatives listed under "Ingredient Substitutes" (page 165-166). You can also add chopped nuts or a little protein powder to the mix for extra protein and flavor.

Nutrition per serving: 109 Calories, 11g Carbs, 6g Fat, 5g Protein, 6g Fiber, 5g Sugar

HIGH-PROTEIN BANANA SOFT-SERVE (SERVES 1)

This dessert hits the spot in the summer. After a late-afternoon run and early dinner, I love to relax with a bowl of Banana Soft-Serve. I add protein powder to keep me from wanting seconds, but you can omit it or add a little Greek yogurt for creaminess. Add some nut butter, nuts or chocolate chips if you like.

½ **frozen banana**

1 tbsp/15 g protein powder (chocolate or vanilla)

3 tbsp/45 ml unsweetened vanilla almond milk

2–3 drops stevia

Place ingredients together in a bowl. Using a food processor or hand blender, combine ingredients until they achieve a smooth consistency, like soft-serve ice cream. Add slivered almonds or chocolate chips for crunch. Want a sundae? Melt some peanut butter in a small dish in the microwave and drizzle on top.

Nutrition per serving: 103 Calories, 16g Carbs, 1g Fat, 9g Protein 3g Fiber, 8g Sugar

SHOPPING LIST
DRIED SPICES AND CONDIMENTS

You need to buy these only once in a while. Go through your cupboards and pantry and check to see which ones you have. If you don't have them already, pick them up. They should last you 1 to 6 months or more.

- Garlic powder
- Cayenne (red pepper)
- Himalayan sea salt
- Allspice
- Cinnamon
- Dijon mustard
- Balsamic vinegar
- Extra virgin olive oil
- Coconut oil
- Hot sauce
- Oat flour
- Flaxseed meal
- Chia seeds
- Brown rice

STAPLES YOU WILL GO THROUGH MORE QUICKLY

Depending on your favorite recipes, these are staples that have a long shelf life but you might run out of them quickly if you are using them frequently. These will probably need to be purchased about once a month.

- Peanut butter
- Steel-cut oats
- Old-fashioned oats
- Stevia drops or packets (I like NuNaturals, sold online and in Whole Foods)
- Protein powder, whey or vegan (I love Vega and Perfect Fit)
- Quinoa
- Raisins
- Laughing Cow light cheese wedges
- Ezekiel bread or other favorite whole-grain brand
- Nonfat chicken broth

ON YOUR LIST EVERY 2 WEEKS

- Almonds
- Cashews
- Seeds such as pepitas
- Frozen mango chunks
- Frozen berries
- Frozen veggies, such as broccoli, asparagus, peppers and onions

- Tuna, unsalted, water-packed
- Sweet potatoes
- Canned pumpkin
- Salsa
- Tomato sauce (fewer than 7g of sugar per half cup/118 g)

ITEMS TO PURCHASE WEEKLY

- 2 lbs/896 g boneless, skinless chicken breasts (6–8 servings)
- 2 lbs/896 g ground turkey (6–8 servings)
- 1 lb/448 g sliced turkey (4 servings)
- 1 lb/448 g shrimp (3 servings)
- 1 lb/448 g flaky white fish (3 servings)
- 1 15.5 oz/427 g can chickpeas or black beans
- 3 lemons
- 4 bananas
- 3 apples
- 2 grapefruit

- 2 bags organic mesclun greens, romaine or baby spinach
- 1 bunch of kale
- 1 cucumber
- 1 medium red onion
- 1 1-lb/448-g bag of baby carrots
- 1 1-lb/448-g bag of celery
- 1 small container of hummus
- 32 oz/950 ml (or more) unsweetened almond milk or other nondairy milk

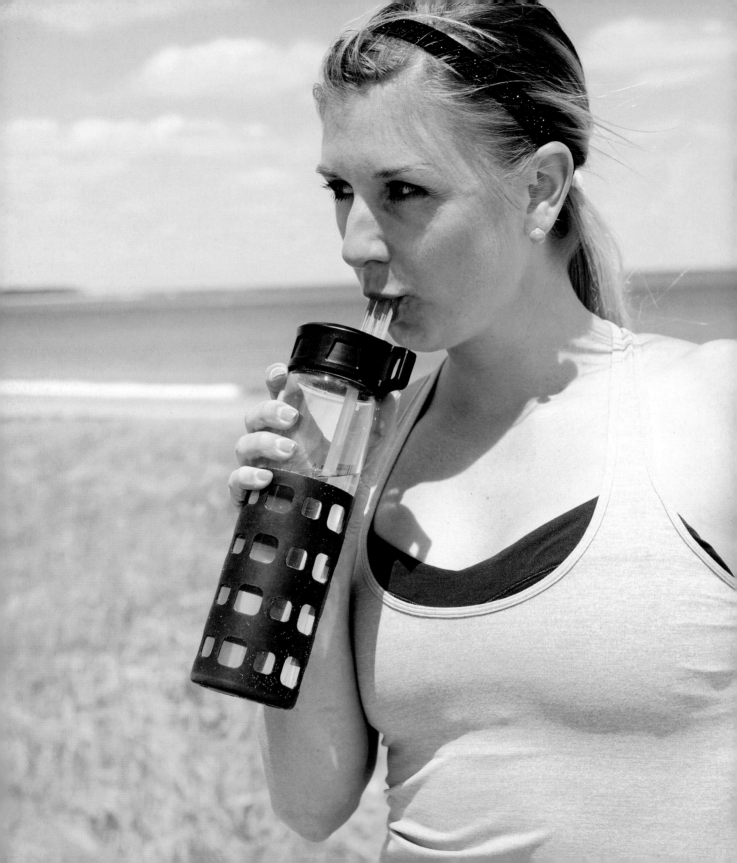

CHAPTER 5

TIME TO DETOX

Between the environment that we live in, the food we put in our mouths and our stressful lives, our bodies have become increasingly toxic. The bad news is that our bodies do not know what to do with many of these chemicals. Often they are stored in the body, which can lead to a variety of ailments that we try to cover up with medicine or ignore altogether. The good news is that for the most part, we can detoxify on our own with a well-rounded, clean diet.

Headaches, bloating, gas, depression, constipation, eczema or psoriasis, fatigue, cravings, compulsive eating, arthritis, asthma, learning disabilities, anxiety, and stomach pains are just a few signs and symptoms of having a toxic body.

When it comes to environmental toxins, they're pretty hard to escape these days. Plastics, cleaning supplies, beauty products, pesticides, heavy metals such as mercury and over-the-counter drugs and prescriptions contribute to the amount of toxins our bodies are exposed to on a daily basis. And that's before we even sit down to eat! You can naturally reduce your toxic load with these tips.

To reduce the amount of environmental toxins your body is exposed to, drink filtered water out of glass bottles. Avoid water bottles and other containers made with bisphenol A (BPA), which has been linked to obesity and kidney and heart disease. BPA is a hormone disruptor and xenoestrogen, which means it mimics estrogen and potentially feeds cancers.

Switch to organic beauty products or do the best you can by avoiding ingredients listed as fragrance or perfume and elements ending with *paraben*. Sixty percent of what we put on our skin is absorbed into our bloodstream, including unsafe chemicals like parabens and phthalates, which disrupt the hormonal system. Phthalates are also estrogen mimickers, a synthetic ingredients added to shampoo, hair gel, nail polish, deodorant and other cosmetics to plasticize the product and give it a lasting scent. It appears on the label often as "fragrance" or "perfume." Europe and Canada have strict regulations on the use of phthalates, but the United States does not. Along with hundreds of more regularly used ingredients, these chemicals have been linked to obesity, birth defects, diabetes, asthma and possibly breast cancer, to name a few. One of my favorite sites to check my products is run by the Environmental Working Group, EWG.org. You can search for your favorite products to find out how toxic they may or may not be.

In addition, the food that we eat is contributing to our toxicity levels. Artificial colors, sulfites, artificial sweeteners, high-fructose corn syrup, hydrogenated oils, BHA/BHT, MSG and heavy metals are or contain chemicals our bodies do not respond to well. You should be able to avoid these if you follow a clean-diet plan, but always read your nutrition labels. Limit packaged foods and minimize exposure to genetically modified corn, soy and sugar. Look for the non-GMO verified label when purchasing these. Produce that is labeled organic is usually a safe bet. The organic label does not necessarily mean a food is more nutrient-dense, but that it has been raised without chemical pesticides, so fewer toxins are going into your body.

As a rule of thumb, if a fruit or vegetable has a thick skin like a banana or an orange, you can get away with conventionally grown. Organic produce can be more expensive, so save your money when buying these foods. But when shopping for foods such as grapes, berries, cherries, peaches, nectarines, apples, bell peppers, lettuces, celery and tomatoes, buy organic if you can afford it, as they have been found to have the highest traces of pesticide residue. And always wash them thoroughly.

When it comes to meat, fish and other animal products, I highly recommend buying organic if you can. They are given access to pasture, direct sunlight, and have freedom to move and fresh air. They also have not been given growth hormones, antibiotics or genetically modified feed. What your food ate is what you eat when you consume it. Other terms to look for are *pastured, vegetarian diet, grass-fed, free-range, cage-free* and *wild-caught.*

Toxins are fat-soluble. Your body requires nutrients such as B vitamins, folic acid, and glutathione to process and eliminate toxins; otherwise, they are stored in your fat cells. For this reason, it's important to eat a nutritious diet and maintain a healthy weight. The more fat you have, the more toxic your body can become if you are not eliminating the toxins.

"Eat the rainbow" to get all the important nutrients that your body needs. Some foods to help you naturally detox include raw tomatoes, spinach, carrots, garlic and grapefruit. Egg yolks are filled with B vitamins. Seeds, nuts, beans, watermelon, apples, avocados and asparagus are also especially great. Cilantro has been shown to help move heavy metals out of your system. Infrequently used fresh herbs and spices, such as burdock, ginger, dandelion and turmeric also help detox the body.

If you believe that you may have a high level of toxicity, first start by making the changes that I suggested above. You may be thinking that you have been eating a pretty healthy diet and don't use any of the products mentioned, but you still have many of the symptoms of toxicity. How can you detox your body?

First, you may have a hidden food allergy. Try an elimination diet like the Virgin Diet to find out. The Virgin Diet identifies the 7 foods most likely to be causing food intolerances in our diets today. Some of these are marketed as "diet foods" and may be causing you to gain weight if your body is sensitive or allergic to them. Next, try a juice, vegan or eat-clean cleanse if you are interested. I've battled sugar cravings my whole life, and after losing 10 pounds for a photo shoot, I thought I'd finally kicked the habit. When Thanksgiving brought the sweet tooth back, I finally decided to try a juice cleanse to see if would help me bounce back and reset my body.

MY JUICE CLEANSE EXPERIENCE

A couple of years ago a friend of mine who lived in New York City asked me about my thoughts on juice cleanses. They were all the rage in the city, with everyone from soccer moms to young professionals looking to get rid of toxins in their bodies, clean out their colons and, they hoped, lose a few pounds. My response: "I don't believe you need to drink juice to detox your body. It has the ability to do it on its own. Just eat clean."

Cleanses and detox diets have become increasingly popular over the past 10 years. Yogis, raw foodists, and vegans were the first to praise their benefits. The low-carb and high-protein dieters laughed at the idea of consuming liquid sugar all day. Why remove the fiber content from fruit and vegetables? Where do you get your protein? Why starve yourself if the weight is going to come right back?

I was one of these people, yet the number of people who kept asking me what I thought about the various cleanses was climbing.

In October 2012 I tried my first green juice and was intrigued. I was on my way out to California to shoot a series of ab workout videos for Lionsgate's YouTube channel, BeFit. I had been eating clean and avoiding sugar, and I felt great, but was nervous that I would look bloated on camera after the cross-country flight. Looking for a solution to make sure things were moving along, I tried an all-veggie green juice at Earth Bar. I felt immediately energized and was surprised to feel full afterward. After that, I had a green juice every day for the duration of my visit.

When I got home to Boston, I started researching juice cleanses and decided to try my first 3-day cleanse after Thanksgiving. My intention was to test whether the cleanse would act like a reset button and to share my experience with my audience. Before the Lionsgate shoot, my diet was near perfect and cravings were rare, but after Thanksgiving my good old sweet tooth came back with a vengeance.

I chose a cleanse that consisted of 3 green juices, 2 citrus-flavored juices and 1 nightly nut milk. You are allowed to eat a quarter of an avocado, some celery or a small salad, but I managed to avoid consuming anything other than the juices, water, tea and a cheat piece of gum, which is not technically allowed. Days 1 and 2 were not bad. I felt good at the end of each day but did struggle to fall asleep at night as a result of hunger. I also dreamed of food, something I had never done before. The third day was difficult. I got pretty light-headed around 9:00 am, but after that was able to finish strong. I could not believe I'd done a 3-day juice cleanse and liked it!

I craved the green juice when I woke up. I wanted only fruits, veggies, nuts and beans. It was strange, to say the least. The biggest change was that I had no desire to drink any coffee. I wanted tea. *To this day, I still prefer tea to coffee.*

Did I lose weight? Yes, but when I say weight, I mean water weight, which comes back on. Did it reset my cravings? You bet. Did I need to drink juice to do this? No, probably not, but here is why I continue to juice.

1. Juicing gives your liver and stomach a break.

2. Juicing eliminates decisions about what to eat, as everything is controlled, which makes it easy to follow and helps prevent cravings.

3. The vitamins that your body absorbs on a juice cleanse assist the body's elimination of toxins and help you restart with a clean slate.

I did not have any odd bathroom experiences, although if you do not regularly eat well, you may have a different experience. I've been told the best time to do a colon cleanse, if you ever want to do one, is right after a juice cleanse.

WHY A JUICE CLEANSE CAN BE DANGEROUS

Cleanses are pretty low in calories and deficient in protein and fat, which your body needs to function. Though you can live on 1,200–1,400 calories for up to 7 days in a row, eating so few calories for a prolonged period will cause your metabolism to slow down. There is very little protein consumed during a juice cleanse. After 7 days, your body asks where the heck the protein went! It starts to take protein from your muscles to function properly. This is not good, especially if you are active. When you begin to eat a normal diet again, you will inevitably gain weight—unless you modify your diet to eat fewer calories for good.

Exercising while doing a juice cleanse is probably not in your best interest. I did light exercise during mine, but my heart rate did not exceed that of a moderate effort. During a 60-minute class, I burned a total of 300 calories. So yes, you can exercise, but do not plan on going to a spin class or training for a marathon while doing one. Opt for a routine that does not include cardio. Yoga is a great option.

JUICING IS *NOT* FOR EVERYONE

Yes, your body can detoxify itself without juicing, but the reason I enjoyed my experience was that I didn't have to go grocery shopping, I didn't have to prepare any meals and the rules were simple. Just drink a juice every 2–3 hours. I'm a pretty impulsive person, and saying no to cupcakes is not my specialty, but when I'm paying good money to detox, it makes saying no pretty easy.

And I enjoyed giving my stomach a break from working overtime to digest all the high-fiber foods I love.

Are you wondering if juices are high in sugar? The sugars are naturally occurring. Though science might suggest that the lack of fiber will cause your blood sugar to spike, it surprisingly does not. The extremely micronutrient-dense juice delivers vitamins and minerals instantly throughout your body, which stimulates the liver and gastrointestinal tract, which helps eliminate toxins and waste.

A few words of caution:

• Beware of beet juice. Some people experience a rare allergic reaction to raw beet juice that causes nausea and vomiting.

• Make sure you drink plenty of water.

• You can try a juice cleanse for 1–7 days. Some people do 14 days, but I can't imagine doing that myself. I found 3 days to be perfect, and even 1 day as a tune-up after a holiday splurge is great.

Bottom line: You don't have to do a juice cleanse to detox your body, but if you do decide to try one, it will reset your body and stop junk-food cravings. Also, after you do a juice cleanse, you reestablish your taste buds' sensitivity. For example, you may find cinnamon adds enough sweetness to your morning oatmeal that sugar is no longer necessary.

When it comes to choosing a juice cleanse, I like going with a local company. The juice should stay fresh for only about 3–4 days. If it stays fresh longer, it has been flash-pasteurized, and there is some debate about whether that's as nutritional as nonpasteurized. Regardless, it must stay cold. I have had a few companies ship me juice from all over the country. They deliver it to your door via UPS or FedEx in the morning, so if you have to go to work, have them deliver it to your workplace if you have a fridge there. If you can't be sure that you will be home when it arrives, you risk missing the shipment and having the juice sit in a hot warehouse all day, which will inevitably cause it to go bad. Ordering from a local juicer will allow you to pick it up or have them drop it off at your house personally at a time you request. I use The Ripe Stuff in Boston, and the owner drops it right off at my apartment the night before I want to begin. You'll also support your local economy and keep your dollars in state. The average cost per day for 6 juices is between $40 and $60. You can usually find a discount online using a coupon code or through a site with flash sales, such as Gilt.

There are a few other cleanses that I support as well. I love the Tone It Up 7-Day Slim Down, Tosca Reno's Eat-Clean Cooler 1 plan, Kris Carr's vegan 21-day Challenge Cleanse, and the Virgin Diet I mentioned earlier.

I do not recommend the Master Cleanse because it lacks many vitamins and nutrients that are required for your body to function healthily and to eliminate toxins and waste.

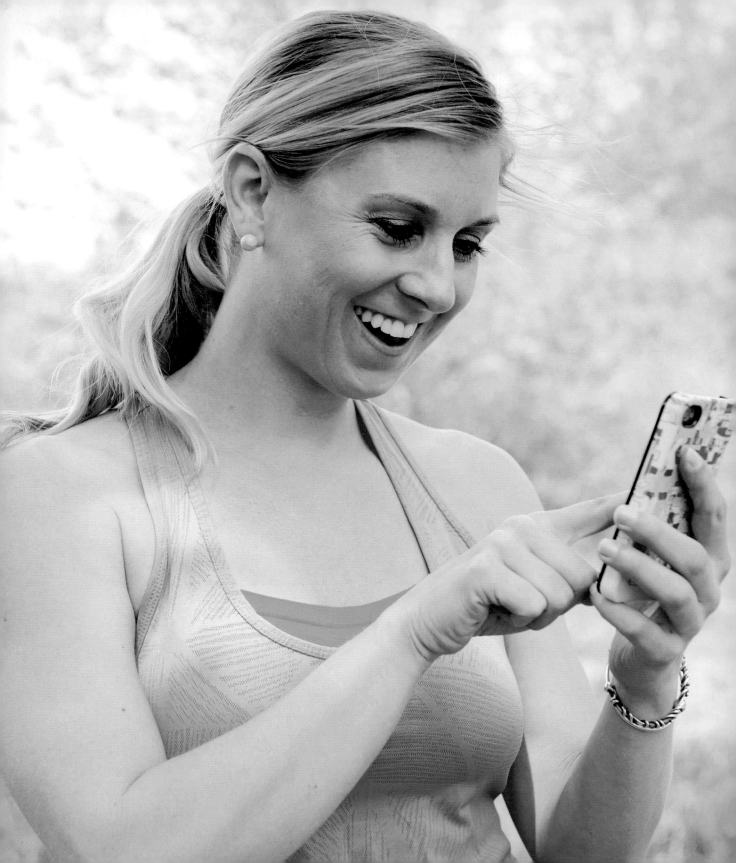

CHAPTER 6

TIME TO BE SOCIAL

If you want to lose weight as an adult, one of the most challenging factors is navigating the social scene without feeling like an outcast. Some of my fondest memories include drinks out with the girls followed by late-night pizza and hangover bagels for breakfast the following morning. When I realized this was not something I enjoyed doing anymore, I thought I might have to become a hermit. Fortunately, you don't have to.

In this chapter we'll discuss some of the most common settings that you will find yourself in and how to make decisions that are consistent with getting skinny again. I am not a certified nutritionist or registered dietician. I am a holistic health coach, and this advice is what helped me achieve my best body.

"CAN I BUY YOU A DRINK?"

First, I command you to learn how to go out, have fun and not have a single cocktail (it doesn't count if you're the designated driver). If you have never done this, you will be amazed that no one cares whether you have an alcoholic beverage in your hand. If you feel more comfortable holding something in your hand, ask for a seltzer water with lime. When you get asked if you want a drink, just say, "No thanks, I'm good." You do not need to explain yourself.

If you are serious about losing weight quickly, alcohol is your enemy. Want to lose the last 5 pounds for your wedding? Don't drink for a month beforehand. Alcohol lowers inhibition and places a focus on immediate gratification, making you forget about the consequences of eating an entire pizza or hooking up with an ex. When you wake up with regret, healthy food and working out are the last things your headache is asking you for.

Alcohol is made of sugar, but it's the not the vodka that is making you gain weight, it's the sugary mixers that you add to it in addition to a lack of portion control.

One of the top 10 questions I get from readers is "What is the best alcoholic drink for me to order if I'm trying to lose weight?"

LIGHT BEER

Honestly, beer is not the devil unless you are gluten-sensitive or have celiac disease. A typical single bottle of light beer has between 90 and 120 calories. It's perfectly portion-controlled for your convenience.

I can hear the moaning already. "It makes me bloated, I don't like the taste . . . blah, blah . . ." If you don't like the taste of beer or how it makes you feel, move on to the next option. If you love the taste of good craft beer, my suggestion is to do your own research. Some *are* light in calories but are not marketed as such. Since craft brews vary by geography, it's up to you to do some digging before heading to the bar or do an inconspicuous Google search on your smart phone. Wheat beers, which are fruity (and most likely purposely geared toward women) are at least 130–170 calories per 12-ounce/350 ml bottle. Among the popular brews that I hear my friends ordering all the time, Blue Moon has 171 calories but Leinenkugel's Summer Shandy has only 130. A bottle is 12 ounces/350 ml, but a pint/475 ml glass, which is usually served when the beer is on tap, will jump the calories in a Blue Moon to 225 per serving.

Two bottles of Michelob Ultra will cost you 190 calories versus 2 Blue Moons on tap for 450 calories.

My personal favorite light beers typically available at most bars include Budweiser Select, Michelob Ultra and Corona Light.

Craft beers that I like and are also pretty low in calories include 21st Amendment Bitter American (132 calories), Harpoon Summer Beer (150 calories), Sam Adams Light (119 calories), Leinenkugel Summer Shandy (130 calories) and Brooklyn Brewery Summer Ale (150 calories). Have a favorite local brewery? Check their website to see how many calories are in each of their beers.

Bottom line: Beer has less sugar than most sodas and juices. If you truly enjoy the taste of craft brews, then have 1 or 2. It's easy to overpour a glass of wine or ounce of liquor, but a bottle of beer is already portion-controlled and takes longer to drink.

WINE

Wine is another great option for the calorie-conscious. I love white-wine spritzers and will mix half a glass of sauvignon blanc with seltzer water. A serving of wine is usually 4–5 ounces/120–150 ml, but many wine glasses these days can hold 3 times that! Like beer, a serving is about 90 to 120 calories, but you will usually be served more, whether you're at a bar or at a friend's house.

Calories in wine will vary depending on the alcohol content. Since wine does not have a nutrition label, to figure out its calories you must look at how much alcohol it contains, also known as the ABV. For a wine with 9–12 ABV, you will get about 110 to 140 calories per serving.

Sparkling wine like Champagne and Prosecco have added sugar for the fermentation process. Opt for brut natural or brut zero, which means very little sugar has been added. A 5-ounce glass will run you about 120 calories per glass. Avoid bottle labeled "doux" because, of all the sparkling wines, these have the most sugar added and are therefore the sweetest.

Dessert wines have the most calories and can run you up to 300 calories per serving. I'd rather have dessert than these any day!

Dry white wines typically have fewer calories than red wines, but red is said to have some heart-healthy benefits, which makes it the top choice of many nutritionists.

There have been many studies on the benefits or lack thereof of alcohol. One of the most talked about says that people who drink red wine tend to live longer. Credit was given to antioxidants found in the skin of red grapes that help prevent heart disease by reducing bad cholesterol and protecting our arteries from damage. However, another study showed that people who drink red wine tend to be wealthier, younger and less likely to smoke and are more physically fit than beer drinkers. When those factors were taken into account, beer and wine drinkers lived just as long as each other.

Red wine does contain beneficial antioxidants, such as flavonoids and resveratrol, that may or may not reduce your chances of getting heart disease. If you are reading this book, chances are you care about your health, so do yourself a favor and drink in moderation.

LIQUOR

Since liquor has the highest ABV, there are a ton of calories in that little shot glass, about the same that come in a full beer or 5 ounce/150 ml glass of wine.

I once knew a guy who was 30 years old and didn't know vodka had calories. I wish I were joking, but I'm not. A shot of tequila has about 100 calories. Yes, in just 1.5 ounces/45 ml, you get the same number of calories that you do in an entire freaking beer! That's why it tastes awful, and if you like to sip vodka or tequila straight, bravo! You are truly unusual. To make these crazy fluids taste halfway decent, you have to add flavor. The cheapest way for a bartender do that is with sugar. Fruit juices and syrups make the medicine go down, right? Thank goodness Bethenny Frankel finally made skinny cocktails convenient to order. Of course, you can try ordering a skinny anything these days at a bar, but here are my standbys, which even the grimiest dive bar will have on hand.

Most vodkas have about 95 to 100 calories per 1.5 ounce/45 ml shot. Here are some of my favorite vodka drinks.

Vodka Soda: Boring but practical and will always be available! Flavored vodkas taste great, but most are made with extra sugar and artificial flavors that make that hangover oh so memorable. Every bartender knows how to make one. Ask for a splash of pineapple juice and lime for your own natural flavor. For a classy spin, ask for a splash of Grand Marnier and extra lemon slices that you can squeeze into the drink.

Ice Pick: In college we used to drink unsweetened iced tea and vodka at Klondike Kate's with a packet of sweetener. I use stevia now, but back then it was Splenda or Equal. Your typical dive bar probably does not have this, but most restaurant bars will. Yes, I take my own sweetener with me to restaurants and coffee shops. Don't judge. Also, don't forget to ask for your slice of lemon!

Bloody Mary: These used to make me cringe, and I still need to be in the mood, but there is nothing better than a spicy Bloody Mary at a hangover brunch. I do not drink more than one, but it's not a bad way to get some veggie vitamins when you aren't feeling so hot.

Skinny Watermelon Margarita: Ask for this at most bars and they should be able to make one for you, even if it's not on the menu. You can also make your own at home with this simple recipe, which makes 2 margaritas, because drinking alone is never fun. Halve the ingredients for a single serving.

Rum is also fairly low-calorie and goes well with low-sugar mixers such as coconut water. Like vodka, the flavored varieties will have some added sugar, giving you a worse hangover if you overdo it. My favorites are the coconut, mango and pineapple rums. Here are a couple of my favorite rum drinks.

SKINNY WATERMELON MARGARITA (SERVES 2)

2 shots clear tequila (3–4 ounces/90–120 ml)

3 limes

2 cups/152 g diced fresh watermelon

Juice the lime. I like to roll them firmly on the countertop first. I cut down the equator and squeeze out as much as I can. Then I poke a fork into the pulp a few times and squeeze again. (You can also use a citrus juicer, which I recommend buying if you plan to start your day with warm lemon water as I do. It costs only about $10 to $14 but will save you time in the morning, and you'll get more juice out of your citrus fruits.) Next, combine the tequila, lime juice and watermelon in a blender. Blend well and serve over ice. Sweetener not needed.

Skinny Colada: Most restaurants do not serve coconut water, so this one is for at home or to take the beach. I have to give credit to Legal Seafood in Boston for inspiring this cocktail. Mix a shot of clear pineapple-flavored rum (such as Parrot Bay) with 4-6 ounces of unsweetened coconut water. You may use mango, coconut or regular rum as well. I like regular coconut water because there are no added sugars; however, for this drink a flavored one such as pineapple coconut water will taste great as well.

Skinny Spring Break Rum Somethin': At a bar and want something sweet without too many calories? Ask for mango-flavored rum with soda water and a splash of pineapple juice. If you don't like sweet drinks, don't get this, but if you're craving that crazy drink special on the menu that costs $15, save your money and calories for later in the night and order this.

There are a few drinks that mix wine and liquor, such as Champagne cocktails and sangria. My favorite Champagne cocktail is made with sparkling wine, soda water and elderflower liqueur, such as St. Germain. I also love a good sangria. Ask if it's made with added sweetener, ginger ale or Sprite. If it is, tell the bartender to make it with soda water instead and skip the extra sugar, since the fruit juice makes it sweet enough. If it's premade, opt for something else, as it can be a calorie disaster: 250 to 300 calories per 6 ounces/180 ml at most chain restaurants.

If you want to drink, make smart decisions. Do not order a Long Island iced tea, piña colada, mudslide, or premixed margarita if you are serious about getting skinny again. Be basic. Order simple.

"WE SHOULD TOTALLY GRAB DRINKS!"

I hear this phrase weekly. Grabbing drinks for 20- and 30-somethings is a great way to network, catch up with friends, meet future husbands and celebrate special occasions. There are, however, alternatives that many people seem to ignore.

Get pretty, not sloshed. Instead of hitting a bar to catch up with a girlfriend and ignore guys who try to hit on you, visit a nail salon together. Depending on your city, it will cost you anywhere from $10 to $40 to get a manicure or pedicure (or both). Not only will it be cheaper than 2 glasses of wine at most restaurants, but you also avoid screaming over the music.

Have lunch instead of dinner. Instead of going out for dinner, meet up with friends for brunch. It's much cheaper and though cocktails are offered, declining a bloody is a sign that you can hold your own and do not need "the hair of the dog that bit you." How mature of you.

Sweat while you gossip. Having a workout buddy is a great way to get motivated to work out but it's also a terrific way to help friends mend broken hearts, solve problems or just bitch to get it all out. This might not sound like a great idea, but for the friend who doesn't know when to stop talking, this might be a good option! You can keep quiet while her stories help pass the time.

Trying out a new studio is also a fun way to get together with a friend. It's easy to bail on a class reservation when you have no one meeting you there. Grab a fresh juice or salad afterward to round out the healthy package.

Forced into a work-related happy hour? If you don't want to drink, grab a soda water with lime and tell the gang you are meeting a friend at the gym afterward but didn't want to miss out on the fun. Ordering a beer is always a good bet at social events that you don't really want to drink at but don't mind having one or two. It will last longer than a glass of wine.

DINING OUT DILEMMAS SOLVED

Going out to eat more than twice a week is a quick way to ruin your hard work toward getting skinny again. I suggest giving yourself two cheat meals a week. While you may be ordering the healthy entrée, really you are still eating 300 more calories than you would be if you were at home! It's not helping you reach your goal at all. I love to go out to eat, which is why I eat most of my meals at home—when I do eat out, I can order what I think sounds good. It's possible to eat well at restaurants, but, still, the egg-white omelet, a seemingly healthy choice, is cooked in pats of butter with veggies sautéed in tablespoons of oil. That omelet just became one of your cheat meals. Don't feel bad about it, but also don't give yourself a pat on the back.

Don't think, though, that if you're going to have a cheat meal, you might as well go all out and order the bacon cheeseburger with fries. That is the exact mentality that is going to prevent you from reaching your goals. A restaurant's idea of healthy is usually my idea of a splurge meal. Be smart about it. If you feel uncomfortably full by the end of a meal, it was a cheat meal.

A consultant and the author of *Never Eat Alone*, Keith Ferrazzi, recommends social dining for networking opportunities and getting ahead in life, but this idea has a huge effect on human dietary behavior. Studies show that how much our dining companion eats at a meal affects how much we eat. When friends go out together, they tend to eat the same amount. One study reported that people who have mostly overweight friends most likely end up overweight themselves. If you dine out with a group, you eat similar amounts even if it's more than you are used to.

However, another study published in October 2012 by the University of Minnesota revealed that social norms have a strong influence on how much we eat, even when it is restrictive behavior. If your friends say no to dessert, you are more likely to say no as well. I'm not asking you to choose your friends on the basis of the scale (that would be ridiculous and I would *never* do that), I am suggesting that you listen to your body and follow your own cues rather than following others' leads.

Here are some ways to keep your eating in check:

- Take breaks while you are eating. It's okay to put down your fork temporarily in the middle of a meal.

- Chew your food thoroughly. During each meal, take the time to really chew at least 3 different mouthfuls 30 times. This helps practice mindfulness. Do you like the taste of what you are eating? How hungry are you still?

- A serving of meat is about the size of your palm. Most restaurants will serve you twice that. Take note to take home half for lunch tomorrow.

- Drink plenty of water 20 minutes before you start eating. Drinking too much water in the middle of your meal may disrupt digestion.

- Before you go to the restaurant, eat a handful of almonds or a small apple. Having a pregame snack will help prevent overordering, digging into the bread basket and impulse decisions.

BUT WHAT SHOULD YOU ORDER?

I love going to tapas restaurants with my friends. Tapas are small plates that are meant for sharing and served family style. Traditionally, they are Spanish cuisine, but many restaurants serve just about anything tapas style.

We typically split a bunch of small plates that are served throughout the night. This style of eating really forces you to check in with your hunger levels. Since the plates are small and no one wants to be rude, everyone takes just a little bit. This forces you to put down your fork during the meal. We keep ordering until we are full. I don't think I've ever left a tapas restaurant uncomfortably stuffed. Since portions are small, you don't have to feel guilty about ordering the less-than-healthy options.

When it comes to making a decision on your own, look for grilled lean proteins and lots of vegetables. Don't be afraid to ask the waiter a few questions about how a dish is prepared. If you are shy or prefer not to bother your server, check out Yelp reviews and pictures of dishes served at the restaurant. These show the portions and can help you see how many veggies the dish is made with.

If the restaurant is part of a chain, go to its website and check out the nutrition facts before you go; all chain restaurants are required to post this information. Living in a city, I rarely go to chains for dinner. I just have to use my best judgment, but luckily the non-chain places are more willing to make substitutions and cook to order.

Steak houses are one of the easiest places to eat clean. Ordering à la carte gives you some freedom to load up on veggies. Grilled asparagus, broccoli, Brussels sprouts, sweet potatoes and even cauliflower are usually available at popular joints. Confused about different cuts of meat? Stick with anything that has *round* or *sirloin* in its name. They are the leanest cuts, meaning they have the most protein. Remember, 4 ounces/112 g is a serving and most places serve twice that. Steak houses also serve healthy fish entrees, which I actually prefer.

My go-to meal at many restaurants is a Greek salad with grilled chicken and dressing on the side. If I'm ever in doubt, it's a safe option that I know I'll enjoy. But don't be fooled; salads these days are not always healthy options. It's common for them to come with bacon, cheese, dried fruit, candied nuts, creamy dressing, fried onions, croutons and more. It's not unusual for them to have more calories than burgers.

If you frequently order salads, look for ones with a vinaigrette and ask the waiter if they have an oil-free alternative. If you want cheese, choose ones with goat or feta cheese. They are typically not made from cow's milk and will prevent you from ingesting hormones and chemicals you don't want. Stick with lean proteins like grilled chicken, fish, organic tofu or legumes. Avoid the sugary add-ins like candied nuts or dried cranberries. Raisins do not have added sugar, so these are okay. Croutons are questionable. I love to make my own at home, but at a restaurant they are just buttery processed breads with zero nutritional value. Choose salads with avocado, undoctored nuts, and olives for heart-healthy fats that will help you feel full. And the more fresh veggies, the better.

Here are some strategies for eating at various types of restaurants.

Mexican: Order fajitas. Skip the cheese and sour cream. Load up on guacamole, salsa and other fresh vegetables. Brown rice and beans are a great side. Use restraint with the margaritas and free chips. Put 5–12 chips on a plate if you can't resist and nibble on those with as much salsa as you want. Guacamole is good for you but is high in calories, so be careful not to overdo it.

Chinese: Buddha's delight is usually steamed veggies with tofu. Order sauces on the side. Chicken teriyaki skewers, baked dumplings and steamed spring rolls are safe bets.

Italian: Start with a salad. I also love steamed mussels in marinara as an appetizer. Order a dish that comes with lots of veggies and lean protein. If you are ordering pasta, ask for gluten-free or whole-grain, if available. Eat all the vegetables and protein first, and then move on to the pasta if you are still hungry. I'm usually full by the time I finish my veggies and protein, mainly because I talk a lot at dinner and this allows me to pace myself.

Sushi: Seaweed salad and 4 to 6 pieces of sushi. Sashimi is the bomb. Use tamari, which is gluten-free, instead of soy sauce. "Spicy" usually indicates that mayonnaise is an ingredient, and "crunchy" means it's fried. Steer clear of those.

Everything else: Lean protein and lots of vegetables. This shouldn't be difficult. You can do it. Listen to your belly. Are you still hungry?

Being a vegetarian or a vegan can be tricky if your dining-out choices are limited. There are an increasing number of veggie-centric spots opening up around the country, though, that even carnivores are raving about. Beware of high-fat sauces made with nuts for a creamy effect. Yes, they're animal-free, but that doesn't mean calorie-free. Want a drink? Try kombucha or fresh green juice for a change.

Many restaurants have their menus online. Look at them and make a plan before you leave the house. Don't allow yourself to change your plan because of a pre-dinner cocktail or what the others at your table order. Don't be afraid to ask your waiter questions and request substitutions.

When it comes to ordering dessert, split one for the table. Never order one just for yourself unless it is your birthday!

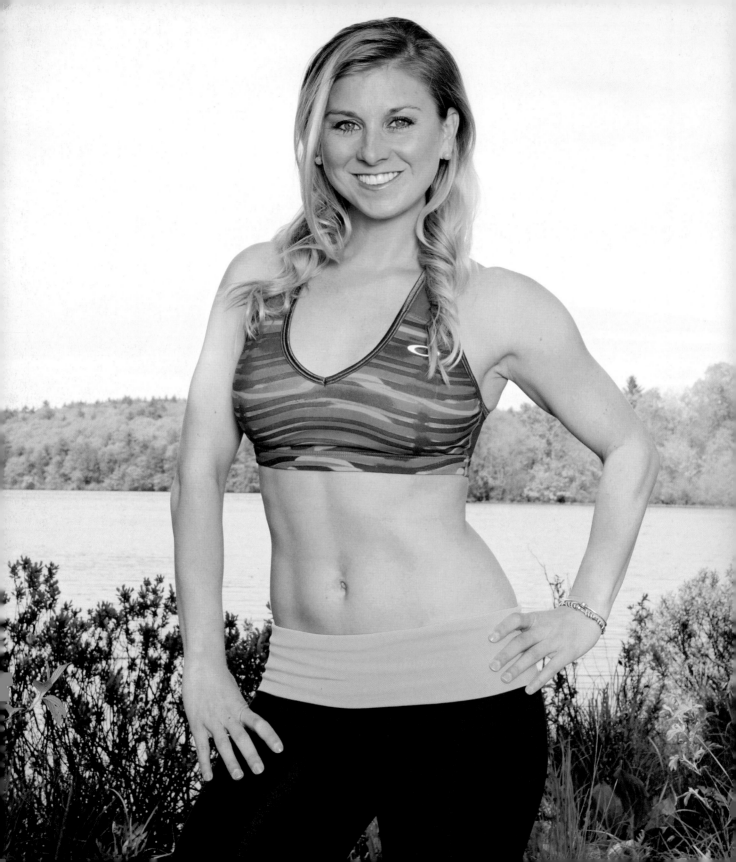

PART THREE

TIME TO LIVE THE FIT LIFE

When it comes to enjoying life, we all need to find a happy balance. I am a party girl at heart who inherited a sweet tooth. If I were to indulge in the two without moderation, I would be unhealthy and unhappy. On the opposite side of the spectrum if I were to completely eliminate dessert or alcohol for good, I would be extremely cranky and unpleasant to be around. I think my blog and YouTube channel resonate with many people because I am not naturally skinny and I do have to work hard for my splurges. These are my tips and tricks that have helped keep me looking fit while celebrating the life that God gave me.

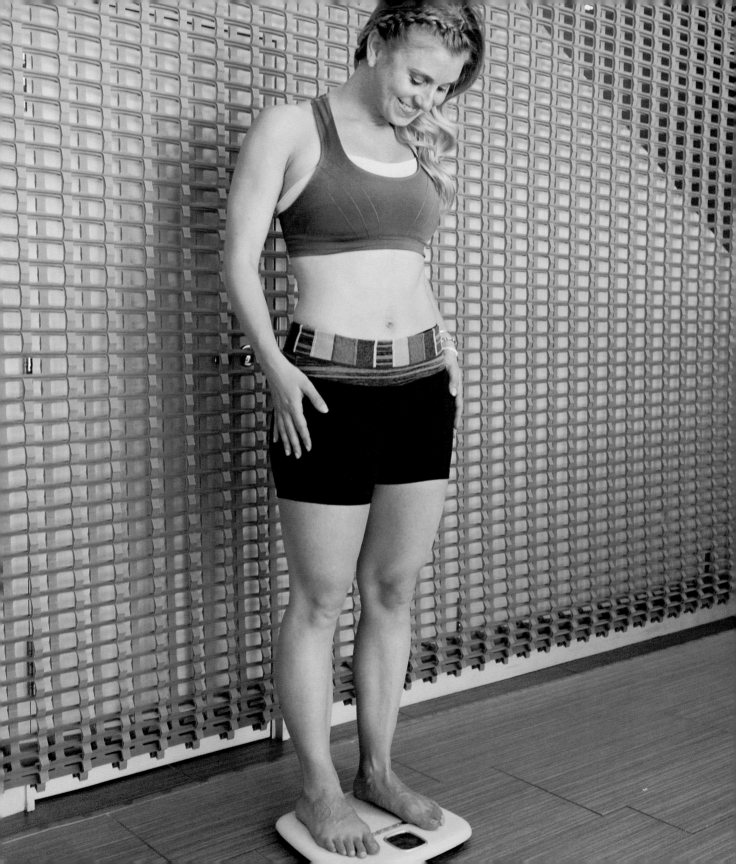

CHAPTER 7

TIME TO GET SKINNY AGAIN

I can remember in college always wanting to weigh 120 pounds/54.4 kg. At 5 feet 4 inches/ 162.5 cm, that would give me a BMI of 20, which is in the "normal" range, 18.5–24.9. I had been a competitive high school athlete and hated my large thighs, which I attributed to years of playing soccer. What I didn't realize at the time was that my legs were pretty much solid muscle and my goal of thinner thighs was unrealistic and unhealthy.

Women need a body fat percentage of at least 10–12% for general good health. But it can be very dangerous to have only this much body fat, as body fat is essential to protect your reproductive organs and bone health. Maintaining a very low body fat for a prolonged period will affect your hormones and your menstrual cycle, which could lead to infertility. If you want to have regular menstrual cycles, you need a body fat percentage of at least 13–17%.

"What about those ladies who compete in bodybuilding figure competitions?" you might ask. They often will drop down to 15% for the week of their event. This weight is not maintained after the competition day itself—trust me. If you meet one of these women during her off-season, you will be shocked at how much her body changes when a competition is not in sight.

For me to be 120 pounds/54.4 kg (my college "goal" weight) with 15% body fat, I would have had to lose an additional 10 pounds/4.5 kg of muscle. Do you see why my original goal wasn't realistic now?

I didn't realize this conclusion until after I trained with a personal trainer for 4 months, twice a week. We planned to do a before-and-after video to show that strength training doesn't create bulky muscles in women. He regularly measured my body fat, and I followed a fairly healthy diet.

I couldn't sleep the night before the final weigh-in because I was so hungry. I wanted the video to be good; I needed to shock the viewer. At 127 pounds/57.6 kg, I measured 14.7% body fat. I was this weight for maybe 1 day because my body was dehydrated. We did this on purpose so that my muscles would "pop" on camera, something the women in figure competitions have mastered for the day of their event as well. We lied on camera to say that I weighed 129 pounds/58.5 kg because we did not want to promote the fact that I had dropped below the recommended 15%. We shot the video and titled it "How I lost 100% of My Excess Body Fat." Currently, the video has over half a million views, but I wish I could add a disclaimer that I gained back 5 pounds/2.3 kg pretty quickly after we finished.

My body weight was too low to sustain my lifestyle. I craved carbs and fat incessantly until my body gained back those extra pounds. At just 5 pounds/2.3 kg heavier, I was able to have my occasional treats and wine while maintaining a weight I was comfortable with.

Female athletes typically have between 15% and 20% body fat, and typical gym enthusiasts have up to 24%. As much as 32% is considered healthy for a female.

Without knowing your body fat percentage, your happy healthy weight may be a challenge to calculate. I'm not a fan of bathroom scales—I find most of them to be very inaccurate. A skin-fold measurement with calipers is one of the most accurate options but needs to be done by a skilled, experienced professional. The most simple option would be to grab a tape measure and calculator.

I've also had mine calculated at one of the top gyms in the United States, Peak Performance in New York City, standing on a highly sophisticated scale with a built-in body-fat monitor that you grip with both hands. If you have access to something like this, then by all means take advantage.

Now that you have a number in mind that you want to achieve, here is the bad news. Sometimes your body doesn't agree with what your mind wants. Enter the phrase "Happy Healthy Weight," your HHW. This weight might not be your ideal, but it's a weight that you can feel confident at while still enjoying some of the indulgence that you love. As I mentioned earlier, when I drop below my HHW, I crave carbs and sugar for a reason. I'm depriving myself, and my body responds by wanting those things even more. This makes the 5-pound/2.3-kg difference unsustainable for very long.

Perhaps you've been at your goal weight before, but your body fought hard to gain back a few pounds through cravings and hunger pangs. This happened to me shortly after I shot the video "How I Lost 100% of My Excess Body Fat." I was at my lowest weight since 9th grade, and all I wanted to do was eat! I was starving. I couldn't sleep, and even when I did, I dreamed of food. After regaining those 5 pounds/2.3 kg, I found that eating clean with a few cocktails on the weekend and the occasional dessert splurge allowed me to fairly easily maintain my HHW. When I say occasional dessert splurge, I don't mean banana "ice cream" or ginger chews, I mean cupcakes and cannolis. At my lowest weight, these treats would send me into a sugar binge, since I was being so restrictive.

I'm also going to let you in on a little secret. When you see a photo of me at a shoot in Malibu or in magazines, I tried really hard to look ripped. It's likely that I lost a few extra pounds of water weight the day of the shoot, which comes back quickly. The photos of me in this book, however, were taken when I was at my HHW! I promise.

Viewers frequently e-mail me asking for help losing weight. Often, the number of pounds they want to lose is very unrealistic. I just want to reach through the computer and preach to them, "You are healthy and thin as is, if you would allow yourself to see it! Don't try to achieve perfection. It doesn't exist."

Start with small, healthy goals. If you have a lot of weight to lose, your HHW may be lower than you think is possible to achieve. You may not discover your HHW right away, but you will with practice.

I got my skinny back while working two jobs. I had just started at NESN and was a waitress on Cape Cod in the summer. In the fall I started working at Diet.com and continued to work at NESN. I would fit in 30-minute workouts at the gym between jobs on days I worked at both or would work out first thing in the morning at 6:30 am. Being busy took my mind off food and eliminated the option of snacking all day.

If you want to know the best time of day to work out to lose weight, the answer it not crystal clear. It really depends on you! I highly recommend working out in the morning, as it sets the tone for the rest of the day. It also allows you to burn a little more fat if you do it first thing on an empty stomach.

For some people who have long commutes or early jobs, this may not be a possibility. Some people are not able to work out with the same intensity in the morning as they might in the afternoon. Afternoon is just as effective; however, things may come up during the day that cause you to bail on your workout if it's scheduled later. You also have more time to make excuses not to do it.

Working out after dinner may disrupt your body's ability to fall asleep easily. That is not true for everyone, though. You have to see what works for you. A workout at a specific intensity will burn the same amount of calories whether it's done morning, noon or night.

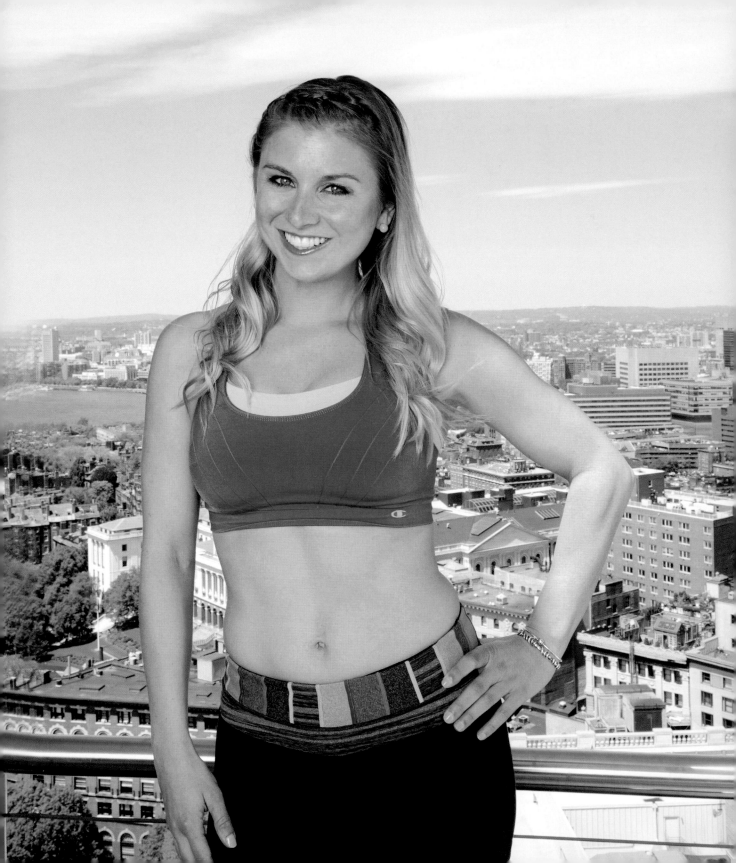

CHAPTER 8

MY STORY

I love what I do, but it was not an easy journey to get where I am today. Unlike a job path towards becoming a police officer or lawyer, mine was not clearly mapped out. Neither YouTube nor Facebook even existed when I entered college!

Growing up, I wanted to be like Katie Couric on *The Today Show,* a broadcast journalist. I would use my family's video camera starting at age 9 to shoot fake news reports, music videos and my own soap operas.

But in college I started to doubt whether my dream job was attainable. I often felt that I was wasting my time. And on top of that, I gained the typical freshmen 15 pounds/68 kg, and I felt terrible about myself. Between soccer and track, I had always been active during high school but without a coach or practice 6 times a week, my fitness routines were not enough make up for my new beer and late-night pizza infatuation.

I loosely followed Weight Watchers to lose the weight. In addition, I was running 5 times a week and strength training two days a week. I got my routines from magazines like *Shape* and *Self*. Jennifer Aniston's body was my inspiration. In my free time, I enjoyed reading health and wellness magazines and experimenting with different recipes. I spent hours grocery shopping, studying products new to the shelves. I began to realize my strong passion for fitness and healthy living.

Two months before graduation in 2006, I was offered a production assistant position at New England Sports Network (NESN), the station of the Red Sox and Bruins. I eagerly accepted this $8/hour part-time position in which my schedule revolved around the Red Sox. I was told that it would turn into a full-time position in the fall, which was a perfect transition, in my opinion, to the "real world."

But September came around and my position at NESN was still part-time, so I began working at Diet.com from 9:00 am to 1:00 pm. I would dash over to the Watertown Boston Sports Club, run on the treadmill for 30 minutes and then head to NESN to work until 11:30 pm or so. My plan was to work at Diet.com long enough that I could build a reel to send to news stations while making my way up at NESN.

My first few videos for Diet.com are incredibly embarrassing if I look at them now. My onscreen awkwardness and lack of sophistication is very apparent. I didn't tell many people what I was doing because I didn't want them to see the videos. A few of my close friends made fun of them, which hurt, but I didn't let that stop me. Gradually, I got more comfortable in front of the camera and the quality began to improve.

Right before Christmas I decided to leave NESN, putting my faith in Diet.com—a job I hid from my friends. As YouTube became more popular, I proposed fitness videos to my boss at Diet.com. I wanted our channel to be something my friends would find helpful. Maybe we could translate the print features into little web videos for people who don't want to spend the money at the newsstand.

After editing and uploading each video to YouTube, I would relentlessly send the video links to blog editors such as Hungry Girl, FitSugar, Perez Hilton, and Jezebel hoping they would feature us. No one would bite. It was frustrating. It seemed that no one knew there were fitness videos on YouTube. So my boss asked me to get a celebrity to star in a video. We both knew this would be a successful way to get people to watch, but I had little hope that someone would say yes. Luckily, my brother worked in Hollywood at a production studio and was able to give me a few agencies' phone numbers.

I started calling B-list celebrities from Massachusetts, hoping they would have some hometown sympathy and would want to help me out. When I called one agency for Maria Menounos I was turned down, but I was then asked if I would be interested in a natural foods chef who was hosting an event called Chef Dance at the Sundance Film Festival. The woman had just finished second on Martha Stewart's *Apprentice,* and now her agents were inviting me to travel around with her to shoot some videos. This woman turned out to be Bethenny Frankel. Needless to say, our videos started getting a lot more attention.

Shortly after, I created my own YouTube channel. Unsure if I wanted to create fitness or health videos, I named it SarahsFabChannel so I could feature anything I deemed fabulous. It was a great idea at 24 years old.

I reached out to Elle Fowler, a popular YouTube beauty guru, after seeing her tweet about losing fat around her midsection. A couple months later, I noticed I was getting hundreds of YouTube emails saying I had new subscribers. I realized that Elle had posted a video and recommended checking out my channel. Suddenly my subscriber box went from 2,000 to 10,000 in a week! This was hands down the defining moment for me: I realized I could do this.

Then I scored a gig with Laughing Cow. Until this point, many companies just wanted to send me free product in exchange for a blog post, and I was struggling to stay afloat. Laughing Cow wanted much more from me, and I had a paying gig! I felt like I had won the lottery. Without a mentor, it was hard to know if I was on the right track, but this helped confirm that I was. I was on cloud nine.

Since then, I've worked with many of my favorite companies, starred in a fitness DVD with Jay Cardiello, shot my own online series with Lionsgate, posed for magazines, traveled all over and made some amazing friends through blogging. It's been almost 4 years since I first created my own YouTube channel, and the journey has been entirely unpredictable but a testament to the fact that hard work does pay off.

Though I have my dream job, it gets harder as I find more success. Fitness, while it doesn't consume my life, is something I dedicate a lot of time to. But I love it, thank God. No matter where you want to end up in life, it's going to take hard work and dedication to get there. But if you're passionate about your goals, it's all worth it in the end.

A lot of my readers and viewers send me questions about starting their own blogs, so here are some things to think about before getting started.

What are you passionate about? Entrepreneurship requires more self-motivation than any other occupation, so you need to be extremely passionate about your goals. If you are not sure, dig into your childhood. What did you love to do while growing up? Another question that be might helpful to answer is: What would you do if money were no object? Personally, I would love to travel the world, exploring different cuisines and learning about health in different cultures.

Pick a name! Select a blog name that is catchy, easy to remember and available on most social media channels. You want your URL, Twitter username, YouTube channel and other profiles to match up so that people can easily find you. Avoid using numbers and something that you might be embarrassed to say out loud at a dinner party with a group of strangers. I did not follow this rule with YouTube and Twitter and still regret it.

Be consistent and regularly post new content. If you are blogging, post at least 2 to 3 times a week. If you are posting videos, upload a new one at least once a week. You want your viewers to read the full article and watch the full video, so keep it interesting, engaging and concise.

Make sure that your blog design is pleasing and easy for readers to navigate. Similarly, make sure that your channel on YouTube is well designed and appropriately conveys what your videos are about. People should be able to quickly find the "About Me" section and links to your social media profiles. Have a friend test your site so you can quickly identify any flaws.

Attend blogging conferences. You don't have to attend all of them, but choose one that focuses on your niche and what you need to improve. From taking pictures to search engine optimization, conferences give you a good understanding of all the components that go into making a blog good. I've also made some good friends at blog conferences. After months of tweeting and corresponding via social media, it's great to finally meet people in person. As my shout-out from Elle shows, you never know who can help you down the road—and vice versa.

Engage with brands on social media. Follow you favorite brands on Twitter and tag them in posts when appropriate. If one of your favorite brands follows you on Twitter, say thank you and let them know how big a fan you are. If you respond to brands frequently, they will notice you. When it comes time to hire someone for a campaign, you will stick out in their minds. Don't be afraid to take a proactive approach.

Be yourself, but always be the best version of it. Having a bad day? Stay away from social media. No one wants to hire a complainer. You are a public person and your personal tweets are being watched. If you think a negative comment is going to benefit your brand or your readers, then share it if you feel obligated. When a company acts irresponsibly or has terrible customer service, I will mention the fact, but only after I've thought carefully about what I will say—never in the heat of the moment. I don't want my followers to get burned, too!

Be professional. If you want this to be your full-time job, do not send a reply e-mail that reads, "OMG. I freakin' love your brand. I can't believe you wanna work with ME!?" First, spell check. Don't use emoticons or emojis or web slang. Know your worth. Don't undersell yourself. Respond to business inquiries in a timely manner and remember to follow up after a phone call to thank them for taking the time to speak with you. Ask if there is anything more you can send. Keep following up if you don't get a response. Corporations take forever to make decisions. Be patient, but don't get excited until you have a contract.

Work for free only on occasion. When I first started, I worked for free in exchange for products. You never know if this might turn into a paid opportunity. I think it's important to offer your services when you are building your numbers, but you first need to build a loyal audience with your recommendations. Your blog should not feature only freebies or paid campaigns. Show off what you buy and use! Be genuine with your opinions. If you hate a free product, tell the company and ask if they would still like you to review it. Most of them will say no thank you and ask for constructive criticism. I turn people down all the time if I don't believe in their product or don't think it fits my brand. Here is the catch with bloggers and free products: If you say no, another blogger is bound to say yes. Your winning argument to get the paid deal is that your audience is bigger, more loyal and more trusting of your opinion because you do fewer freebie reviews. You have to build this trust first, though!

There is plenty of room at the top. It's easy to compare yourself to others and feel bad about yourself. Don't do this! It's negative energy that accomplishes nothing. No one can share what you have to offer in the exact same voice. We are all different. What makes you special? Keep reminding yourself of your message and your goals. Stick with them and stay true to them. Don't let someone else's success derail your energy and passion. We may not travel the same path, but it's possible to end up at the same destination of greatness. Remember, we are always a work in progress.

If you want to create your dream job, go out and do it! Stop procrastinating. There is no right or wrong way to go about it. My entire life was preparing for this job, from making movies when I was a kid to my lifelong love for staying active and healthy. It's just something I am great at. So tell me, what are you prepared to be great at?

RESOURCES

Ansell, Karen. "Drinking Alcohol to Shrink?" *Women's Health,* September 2010, http://www.women-shealthmag.com/weight-loss/alcohol-drinking-and-weight-loss-tips.

Heid, Markham. "Is Wine Really Healthier Than Beer?" *Men's Health News,* December 29, 2011, http://news.menshealth.com/is-wine-really-healthier-than-beer/2011/12/29/.

Howland, Maryhope, Jeffrey M. Hunger, and Traci Mann. "Friends Don't Let Friends Eat Cookies: Effects of Restrictive Eating Norms on Consumption among Friends." *Appetite* 59, no. 2 (October 2012): 505–9, http://www.sciencedirect.com/science/article/pii/S0195666312002255.

Kolata, Gina. "Obesity Spreads to Friends, Study Concludes." *New York Times,* July 25, 2007, http://www.nytimes.com/2007/07/25/health/25iht-fat.4.6830240.html?pagewanted=all&_r=0.

Mifflin, M. D., St Jeor, S. T., et al. "A New Predictive Equation for Resting Energy Expenditure in Healthy Individuals." *American Journal of Clinical Nutrition* 51, no. 2 (1990): 241–47, http://ajcn.nutrition.org/content/51/2/241.abstract.

Neergaard, Lauren. "Study: 10 Minutes of Exercise, Hour-Long Effects." *Boston Globe,* June 1, 2010, http://www.boston.com/news/education/higher/articles/2010/06/01/study_10_minutes_of_exercise_hour_long_effects/.

Sotos, Maryelaine. *Detoxification: A Daily Practice of Nourishment and Renewal.* Stockbridge, Mass.: Kripalu Center for Yoga and Health.

Willis, Leslie H., et al. "Effects of Aerobic and/or Resistance Training on Body Mass and Fat Mass in Overweight or Obese Adults." *Journal of Applied Physiology* 133, no. 12 (2012): 1831–37, http://jap.physiology.org/content/113/12/1831.abstract.

ACKNOWLEDGMENTS

I would like to acknowledge my unconditionally loving parents, brother and sister. My mother for piquing my interest in the world of health and nutrition, my father for supporting me and encouraging me to pursue my athletic talents by letting me try every sport imaginable starting at a young age, my brother for inspiring me to follow my dreams and my sister for helping me get through the most challenging years of my career by being my protector, confidant and best friend.

Mom, you inspired me to educate myself about nutrition from an early age. Even at my advanced age of 29, you're still my first phone call when something goes wrong, and I hope it stays that way. Thank you for always believing in me and making me feel like I was special.

Dad, I know how proud of me you are and it means the world. Despite the fact that I write my blog for young women, I love that you read it and are able to take away little things to help improve your own health. Thank you for passing along your running genes to me.

Mike, while we may be 8 years apart, you've been one of my strongest role models. Moving out to LA to pursue your dream is something I will always admire you for. You taught me how to use my first camera in 4th grade and later showed me the ropes of the entertainment industry. Lane and your hospitality never goes unnoticed when I come to visit. I promise never to overstay my welcome.

Mary, I'm not sure I would be where I am today had you not offered me a place to stay right out of college. I probably would have moved to New York to live with my college friends and never entered the YouTube world that started my career. Having a sister who is also a best friend is a gift that I will never take for granted.

Roomie/George, thanks for putting up with the crazy. You help make me the best version of myself, and for that my career is grateful. Thank you for supporting me and helping me grow my business despite your lack of social media interests. Love you.

I would also like to give a giant shout-out and thank-you to the following people:

Mike D, for reminding me that there is always room at the top and inspiring me to become a personal trainer.

Stephen Cabral, for showing me what it's like to be an educated and passionate personal trainer who never stops learning.

Jay Cardiello, for believing in me and helping me network in this very small industry.

Mike Zhang, for knowing back in 2006 that YouTube was going to be as successful as it is today.

Coach Buck, Mr. Astley, Ms. Willis and the rest of my high school coaches, for teaching me how to take criticism and strive to be the best. I now realize what a slacker I must have been, but I learned that quitting was never an option despite conflict with the ones in charge.

Katrina, for being the kind person that you truly are, and reminding me to surround myself with positive and successful people. I don't think Kitty Kat and Sarah from Hoover High had any idea what the future held. Thank you for your and Karena's continued support. I love the Tone It Up community and being a part of it. You're both an inspiration for women, especially business owners.

Cassey and Bex, for being genuine friends in a competitive industry. It's a small circle we work in, and I'm thankful I can call you both friends.

My blog readers, YouTube viewers and fans—without you guys, I would be jobless. Thank you from the bottom of my heart. This book is truly for you.

Thank you to The Ripe Stuff Cleanse, Recycle Studio and The Bar Method Boston for helping me get into cover-girl shape.

Lastly, thank you to Page Street Publishing for helping me put together a book that I wish I had been given while first entering college. It's been a dream to become a published author that you have helped make into a reality. I'm excited to share it with my fans and the rest of the world. Thank you for giving me this opportunity.

Indoor gym shots were taken at the residences at 45 Province in Boston.

Sarah is wearing Oakley Women, Lululemon, DA Active, Reebok, Champion, Lorna Jane, and Sparkly Soul and Kitsch hair ties in the images.

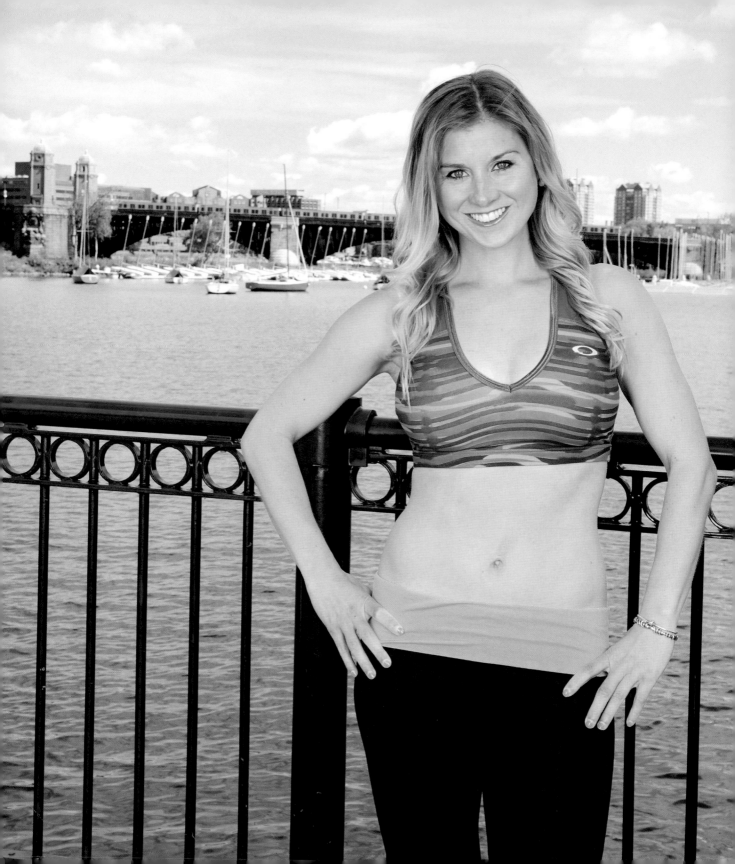

ABOUT THE AUTHOR

Sarah Dussault is one of the most frequently viewed fitness personalities on YouTube. She has produced over 750 videos, earning more than 120 million total views. Since 2006 Sarah has pioneered the YouTube channel for Diet.com, DietHealth, as the senior video producer. From Bethenny Frankel to Ellie Krieger, Dussault has worked with some of the most influential names in the health industry.

She created her own channel, SarahsFabChannel, in 2008 and began blogging shortly thereafter at SarahFit.com. As a full-time blogger, she started out producing, hosting, filming and editing all her own videos.

In 2012 she was named by *Teen Vogue,* FabFitFun and Mashable as one of the top YouTube fitness gurus to follow. She has appeared in various national publications, including *Women's Health, Men's Health, Shape* and *Glamour.*

Sarah has worked and continues to work with many national brands, including Target, Lionsgate, Oakley, PopChips, Laughing Cow, Gatorade, Udi's Gluten Free, Hain Celestial, Polar and more.

Sarah appears in the JCore Body DVD series and infomercial starring Jay Cardiello, a contributing editor to *Shape,* as well as the Six-Pack Abs series produced by Lionsgate's BeFit YouTube channel.

Sarah is a certified personal trainer through the ACSM and trains clients privately in Boston. She is also a certified holistic health coach and Institute of Integrated Nutrition graduate. She earned her bachelor's degree from the University of Delaware studying broadcast journalism.

INDEX

21st Amendment Bitter American, 197

A

ab exercises
  forearm plank, 121, 122
  to lift your butt, 129–137
  physioball jackknifes, 121, 124
  physioball pikes, 121, 126
  scissors, 121, 128
  shin slaps, 121, 125
  teasers, 121, 127
  ten-minute workout for, 121–128
  toe touches, 121, 123
agave nectar, 166
alcohol, 196–197
allergies, 190
allspice, 186
almond butter, 184
almond meal, 166
almond milk, 162, 165, 187
  Chia Pudding, 183
  Energy Balls, 175
  Fruit and Nut Fit Granola Bars, 176
  High-Protein Frozen Banana Soft-Serve, 185
  Instant Pumpkin Pie Mousse, 184
  Peanut Butter and Jelly Time Smoothie, 169
  Protein Pancake, 167
  Tropical Green Smoothie, 168
almonds, 187
  Fruit and Nut Fit Granola Bars, 176
amaranth flour, 166
Aniston, Jennifer, 211
apple, 162
apples, 187
Apprentice, 212
arm circles, 70
arm-toning exercises
  bicep curls to shoulder presses, 144, 145
  high-to-low planks, 144, 148
  plank rows with t-twists, 144, 146–147
  push-ups, 144, 151
  ten-minute workouts for, 144
  triceps dips, 144, 150
  upright rows, 144, 149
asparagus, 164, 187
at-the-gym stretch sequence, 102
Au Bon Pain, 162
avocados, 161
  Summer Quinoa Salad, 173

B

bagels, 161
ball-pass crunches, 89, 94

balsamic vinegar, 174, 186
bananas, 162
  Fruit and Nut Fit Granola Bars, 176
  High-Protein Frozen Banana Soft-Serve, 165, 185
  Post-Workout On-the-Go Protein Muffins, 170
  Protein Pancake, 167
  Tropical Green Smoothie, 168
basal metabolic rate (BMR), 156
beans, 161, 164, 187
beef, 164
beer, 196–197
beets, 164
bell peppers, 187
  Summer Quinoa Salad, 173
bent-over rows, 74, 79
berries, 161, 164, 187
bicep curl balances, 74, 76
bicep curls to shoulder presses, 144, 145
bicycles, 138, 143
Black Eyed Peas, "Pump It," 64
"Bleeding Love" (Lewis), 64
blogging, 213
Bloody Mary, 198
Blue Moon, 196
blueberries, 170
body fat, 207–208
body-weight tri-set, 18–19
Boston Sports Club, 211
bosu ball push-ups with overhead press, 75, 80–81
breakfast, 161
  eating out, 161
  Kale and Quinoa Frittata, 161, 171
  Peanut Butter and Jelly Time Smoothie, 169
  Post-Workout On-the-Go Protein Muffins, 170
  Protein Pancake, 161, 167
  Tropical Green Smoothie, 161, 168
broccoli, 164, 187
Brooklyn Brewer Summer Ale, 197
brown rice, 186
brown rice sushi, 162
Brussels sprouts, 164
Budweiser Select, 196
Buffalo Turkey Meatloaf, 164, 182
butternut squash, 164, 181
butt-lifting exercises
  hamstring curls with exercise ball, 129, 134–135
  single-leg hip lifts, 129, 130
  single-leg squats, 129, 132–133
  sumo squat series, 129, 136–137
  ten-minute workouts, 129–137
  weighted donkey kicks, 129, 131

C

calf foam roll, 104
"Call on Me" (Prydz), 64
calories, 156–157
carbs, 164
Cardiello, Jay, 213
cardiovascular exercise, 11, 12
  core twist jabs, 51, 61
  dance classes, 96
  double squat jumps, 51
  double-squat jumps, 59
  elliptical machines, 96
  Flat Intervals, 101
  forward jumping jacks, 51, 60
  froggers, 41, 49
  get quick and burn fat! 62
  gym-based exercises, 96–101
  at home, 40–65
  hover jacks, 41, 42
  indoor bikes, 96
  interval ladder workout, 100
  interval songs, 64
  jog in place, 51, 52
  jump lunges, 41, 43
  jump rope with oblique twists, 51, 54
  Minute to Win It, 64
  mountain climbers, 41, 44
  oblique burpees, 41, 46–47
  oblique reach and pull, 51, 58
  in-and-out static jump squats, 51, 56
  outdoor running routines, 62–65
  rainy-day 20-minute high intensity interval training (HIIT) workout, 40–50
  rate of perceived exertion (RPE), 98, 99, 100, 101
  side-to-side ninja twists, 51, 55
  single-leg standing crunches, 51, 57
  speed skaters, 41, 48, 51, 53
  speed squats, 41, 50
  Speedy Interval Workout, 98–99
  spinning, 96
  stair-climber, 98
  thirty-minute Plyo-Barre cardio routine, 51–61
  treadmills, 96
  twisting uprights, 41, 45
  Zumba, 96
carrots, 162, 187
cashew butter, Instant Pumpkin Pie Mousse, 184
cashews, 187
cat cow, 68
cayenne, 186
celery, 162, 187
  Buffalo Turkey Meatloaf, 182

Champagne, 198
cheese, 164, 178, 186
    Low-Carb Turkey Wrap, 174
Cheesy Butternut Squash Quinoa, 164, 181
Chef Dance, 212
chest opener, 70
chest presses on physioball, 74, 78
Chia Pudding, 165, 183
chia seeds, 161, 186
    Chia Pudding, 165, 183
    Peanut Butter and Jelly Time Smoothie, 169
chicken, 161, 164, 187
    Buffalo Turkey Meatloaf, 182
    Chicken Salad, 162
    Green Goddess Chicken Salad, 172
    Salsa Chicken, 177
    Salsa Chicken Mexican Salad, 164, 178
    Salsa Chicken Quesadilla, 162
chicken broth, 186
Chicken Salad, 162
chickpeas, 187
cinnamon, 184, 186
clementines, 164
cobra, 67
cocktails, 198
coconut flakes, 161
    Chia Pudding, 183
coconut flour, 166
coconut oil, 186
coconut water, 198
    Skinny Colada, 198
college students, 165
core twist jabs, 51, 61
Corona Light, 196
Cosi, 162
cottage cheese, 161, 164
Couric, Katie, 211
craft beers, 197
cucumbers, 187

D
dance classes, 96
depression, 13
Designer Whey, 166
dessert, 165
    Chia Pudding, 165, 183
    High-Protein Frozen Banana Soft-Serve, 165, 185
    Instant Pumpkin Pie Mousse, 165, 184
detoxification, 189–193
diet, 153–187
Diet.com, 211–212
Dijon mustard, 186
dinner, 164–165
    Buffalo Turkey Meatloaf, 164, 182
    Cheesy Butternut Squash Quinoa, 164, 181
    Eggplant Pasta, 164, 179
    Salsa Chicken, 177
    Salsa Chicken Mexican Salad, 164, 178

    Salsa Chicken Quesadilla, 178
    Sweet Potato Fries, 164, 180
disease prevention, 13
"Dog Days Are Over" (Florence and the Machine), 64
double-squat jumps, 51, 59
downward dog, 67, 68
downward dog split, 67
dried fruits, 176
drinking, 196–197
drinks
    Bloody Mary, 198
    Ice Pick, 198
    Skinny Colada, 198
    Skinny Spring Break Rum Somethin', 198
    Skinny Watermelon Margarita, 198
    Vodka Soda, 198
dumbbell ball v-ups, 88
dumbbell drags, 138, 142
dumbbell swings, 75, 82
dumbbell v-ups, 75
Dunkin' Donuts, 161
Dussault, Sarah, 211–214

E
eating clean, 156
eating out, 195–203
    Chinese restaurants, 202
    Italian restaurants, 202
    Mexican restaurants, 202
    sushi, 202
eating right
edamame, 162
egg whites, 161, 165
eggplant, Eggplant Pasta, 164, 179
Eggplant Pasta, 164, 179
eggs, 161, 162, 165
    Buffalo Turkey Meatloaf, 182
    Kale and Quinoa Frittata, 161, 171
elliptical machines, 96
endorphins, 13
Energy Balls, 164, 175
energy bars, 164
English muffins, 165
entrepreneurship, 213–214
exercise, benefits of, 13
exercise enthusiasts, 12
Ezekiel bread, 161, 162, 165, 186

F
Fatboy Slim, "Rockafeller Skank," 64
Ferrazzi, Keith, 201
figure-four stretch, 108
fish, 164, 187
fitness personality, 12
fitness schedule, 11–14, *12*
    creating, 11
    how many days to work out, 13
Flat Intervals, 101

flaxseeds, 161
flaxseed meal, 170
flexibility training, 11
Florence and the Machine, "Dog Days Are Over," 64
flour, 166
fold over, 67
food allergies, 190
forearm plank, 121, 122
forward fold-over triangle, 69
forward jumping jacks, 51, 60
forward leg lift toe taps, 112
forward leg-lift toe taps, 115
Fowler, Elle, 212, 213
Frankel, Bethenny, 198, 212
french fries, Sweet Potato Fries, 164, 180
frittatas, 161
    Kale and Quinoa Frittata, 171
froggers, 41, 49, 112, 118
fruit, 161, 176
Fruit and Nut Fit Granola Bars, 164, 176
fudge, 165
Furtado, Nelly, "Maneater," 64

G
garlic powder, 186
Get Quick and Burn Fat! 62
gluten-free flour, 166
granola bars, Fruit and Nut Fit Granola Bars, 164, 176
grapefruit, 187
Green Goddess Chicken Salad, 172
greens, 162, 187
gym memberships, 12, 13
gym rats, 12
gym-based exercises, 73–109
    cardiovascular exercise, 96–101
    strength training, 74–95
    stretching, 102–109
gym-free frugalistas, 12

H
hamstring curls with exercise ball, 129, 134–135
hamstring foam roll, 103
hamstring stretch, 68, 108
happy baby dance, 112, 119
Happy Healthy Weight (HHW), 208–209
Harpoon Summer Beer, 197
high intensity interval training (HIIT) workouts, 40–50
high knees, 112, 117
high lunge, 69
high plank, 67
high-intensity workouts, 111–151
High-Protein Frozen Banana Soft-Serve, 165, 185
high-to-low planks, 144, 148
Himalayan sea salt, 186
hip flexor stretch, 68, 106

home-based exercises, 17–71
    cardiovascular exercise, 40–65
    outdoor running routines, 62–65
    rainy-day 20-minute high intensity interval
        training (HIIT) workout, 40–50
    strength training, 18–39
    stretching, 66–70
    yoga poses, 66–70
honey, 166
    Energy Balls, 175
hot sauce, 186
    Buffalo Turkey Meatloaf, 182
Houston, Whitney, "I Wanna Dance with
    Somebody," 64
hover jacks, 41, 42
hummus, 162, 164, 187
    No-Chop Healthy Tuna Salad, 172
    Simple Homemade Salad Dressing, 174

I

"I Made It" (Rudolf), 64
"I Wanna Dance with Somebody" (Houston), 64
Ice Pick, 198
in-and-out static jump squats, 51, 56
inchworm triceps push-ups, 29, 30–31
indoor bikes, 98
ingredient substitutes, 165–166
ingredients, 186–187
inner thigh stretch, 107
Instant Pumpkin Pie Mousse, 165, 184
interval ladder workout, 100
interval running routines, 62–65
interval songs, 64
IT band foam roll, 104

J

jalapeño peppers, Salsa Chicken Mexican Salad,
    178
Jay Robb, 166
"Jetsetter" (Morningwood), 64
jog in place, 51, 52, 112, 113
juice cleanses, 191–193
jump lunges, 41, 43
jump rope with oblique twists, 51, 54

K

kale, 161, 164, 187
Kale and Quinoa Frittata, 161, 171
Karr, Chris, 193
keg-stand shoulder presses, 29, 36
kick-downs, 29, 39
Kris Carr's 21-day Challenge Cleanse, 193

L

lat foam roll, 106
lateral pull-downs, 89, 90
Laughing Cow cheese, 178, 186, 212
leg circles, 29, 35
leg lifts, reverse plank with, 24

Legal Seafood, 198
Leinenkugel, 197
lemons, 187
lentils, 164
lettuce, 187
    Salsa Chicken Mexican Salad, 178
Lewis, Leona, "Bleeding Love," 64
Lionsgate, 213
liquor, 198
Long Day, 71
love handle exercises
    bicycles, 138, 143
    dumbbell drags, 138, 142
    Russian twists, 138, 141
    side plank elbow-to-knee kisses, 138, 139
    spiderman crunches, 138, 140
    ten-minute workouts for, 138
low lunge, 68
Low-Carb Turkey Wrap, 162, 174
low-lunge hip opener, 69
lunch, 161–162
    Chicken Salad, 162
    eating out, 162
    Green Goddess Chicken Salad, 172
    Low-Carb Turkey Wrap, 162, 174
    No-Chop Healthy Tuna Salad, 172
    Salsa Chicken Quesadilla, 162
    Summer Quinoa Salad, 162, 173

M

"Maneater" (Furtado), 64
mangos, 187
    Tropical Green Smoothie, 168
march in place with swinging arms, 66
Master Cleanse, 193
meals, 157–187
    breakfast, 159, 161
    eating out, 195–203
    how many to eat, 157
    meal prep tips, 158–159
    workouts and, 157–158
meatballs, meatless, 164
meatloaf, 164, 182
memory, 13
Menounos, Maria, 212
mesclun greens, 187
Michelob Ultra, 196
milk, 187. See also almond milk
Mini Babybel cheese, 164, 165
mini-pizzas, 165
minute to win it, 64
miso soup, 162
Morningwood, "Jetsetter," 64
mountain climbers, 41, 44, 112, 120
mountain pose, 67
muffins
    On-the-Go Protein Muffins, 161
    Post-Workout On-the-Go Protein Muffins, 170

N

New England Sports Network (NESN), 211, 212
No-Chop Healthy Tuna Salad, 162, 172
nondairy milk, 187
NuNaturals, 166
nut butter, Instant Pumpkin Pie Mousse, 184
nuts, 161, 187
    Chia Pudding, 183

O

oat flour, 166, 186
    Energy Balls, 175
    Fruit and Nut Fit Granola Bars, 176
oatmeal, 161
oats, 186
    Buffalo Turkey Meatloaf, 182
    Fruit and Nut Fit Granola Bars, 176
    Post-Workout On-the-Go Protein Muffins, 170
oblique burpees, 41, 46–47
oblique reach and pull, 51, 58
olive oil, 161, 164, 186
omelets, 161
onions, 187
    Buffalo Turkey Meatloaf, 182
    Summer Quinoa Salad, 173
On-the-Go Protein Muffins, 161
opposite-arm-and-leg supermans, 29, 38
orange, 162
organic foods, 190
outdoor running routines, 62–65

P

pancakes, Protein Pancake, 161, 167
Panera Bread, 162
parsley, Green Goddess Chicken Salad, 172
pasta, Eggplant Pasta, 164, 179
pasta sauce, low-sugar, 179
Peak Performance, 208
peanut butter, 162, 165, 186
    Energy Balls, 175
    Instant Pumpkin Pie Mousse, 184
    Peanut Butter and Jelly Time Smoothie, 169
Peanut Butter and Jelly Time Smoothie, 169
peanut flour, 166
pepitas, 187
Perfect Fit, 166
personal story
physioball chest stretch, 109
physioball jackknifes, 75, 86, 121, 124
physioball pikes, 121, 126
physioball side crunches, 75, 87
pineapples, 168
piriformis foam roll, 103
pizzas, 165
plank, 18, 19
plank rows with t-twists, 144, 146–147
plank with single leg lifts, 29, 37

plyometric movements, 51–61
    core twist jabs, 51, 61
    double squat jumps, 51
    double-squat jumps, 59
    forward jumping jacks, 51, 60
    jog in place, 51, 52
    jump rope with oblique twists, 51, 54
    oblique reach and pull, 51, 58
    in-and-out static jump squats, 51, 56
    side-to-side ninja twists, 51, 55
    single-leg standing crunches, 51, 57
    speed skaters, 51, 53
pork, 164
Post-Workout On-the-Go Protein Muffins, 170, *170*
Pret a Manger, 162
protein, 161, 164
protein bars, 164
Protein Pancake, 161, 167
protein powder, 161, 165, 166, 186
    Energy Balls, 175
    Fruit and Nut Fit Granola Bars, 176
    High-Protein Frozen Banana Soft-Serve, 185
    Post-Workout On-the-Go Protein Muffins, 170
    Protein Pancake, 167
    Tropical Green Smoothie, 168
protein shakes, 162
Prydz, Eric, "Call on Me," 64
"Pump It" (Black Eyed Peas), 64
pumpkin, 187
    Instant Pumpkin Pie Mousse, 165, 184
push-ups, 18, 27, 144, 151

Q
quad stretch, 68
quadriceps foam roll, 105
quesadillas, 162, 178
quinoa, 161, 164, 186
    Cheesy Butternut Squash Quinoa, 164, 181
    Kale and Quinoa Frittata, 171
    Summer Quinoa Salad, 162, 173

R
rainy-day 20-minute high intensity interval
   training (HIIT) workout, 40–50
raisins, 186
rate of perceived exertion (RPE), 98, 99, 100
    cardiovascular exercise, 100, 101
recommendations, applying, 12
red onions, 187
    Summer Quinoa Salad, 173
Reno, Tosca, 193
resistance exercises, 11, 12
reverse lunges with arm reach, 112, 114
reverse plank, 18
    with leg lifts, 24
The Ripe Stuff, 193
roadmap
"Rockafeller Skank" (Fatboy Slim), 64
romaine lettuce, 187

rosemary, Cheesy Butternut Squash Quinoa, 181
Rudolf, Kevin, "I Made It," 64
rum, 198
    Skinny Colada, 198
    Skinny Spring Break Rum Somethin', 198
running routines, 62–65
Russian twist with dumbbell, 75, 85
Russian twists, 138, 141

S
sage, 181
salad dressing, 161–162
    Simple Homemade Salad Dressing, 174
salads
    Chicken Salad, 162
    Green Goddess Chicken Salad, 172
    No-Chop Healthy Tuna Salad, 172
    Salsa Chicken Mexican Salad, 164, 177
    Simple Homemade Salad Dressing, 174
    Summer Quinoa Salad, 162, 173
salmon, 164
salsa, 177, 178, 187
Salsa Chicken, 177
Salsa Chicken Mexican Salad, 164, 178
Salsa Chicken Quesadilla, 162, 178
Sam Adams Light, 197
sangria, 198
SarahsFabChannel, 212
sashimi, 162
scissors, 121, 128
seated low rows, 89, 91
seaweed salad, 162
seeds, 187
seitan, 164
self-confidence, 13
self-esteem, 13
shin slaps, 121, 125
shopping list, 186
shrimp, 164, 187
side lunge relevés, 112, 116
side lunges, 18, 21
side plank elbow-to-knee kisses, 138, 139
side-crunch v-sits, 29, 32
side-plan reach throughs, 18, 28
side-to-side ninja twists, 51, 55
Simple Homemade Salad Dressing, 174
single-leg deadlifts, 75, 84
single-leg hip lifts, 18, 20, 129, 130
single-leg squat toe raises, 18, 22–23
single-leg squats, 129, 132–133
single-leg standing crunches, 51, 57
Skinny Colada, 198
Skinny Spring Break Rum Somethin', 198
Skinny Watermelon Margarita, 198
sliding reverse lunges, 29, 33
sliding side lunges, 29, 34
smoothies, 162, 166
    Peanut Butter and Jelly Time Smoothie, 169
    Tropical Green Smoothie, 161, 164, 168

snacks, 162, 164
    Energy Balls, 164, 175
    Fruit and Nut Fit Granola Bars, 164, 176
    Tropical Green Smoothie, 164
social eating and drinking, 195–203
social media, 214
spaghetti squash, 164
speed skaters, 41, 48, 51, 53
speed squats, 41, 50
speedy interval workout, 98–99
spiderman crunches, 138, 140
spinach, 187
    Tropical Green Smoothie, 168
spinning, 96
sprouts, 174
squash, 164
    butternut squash, 164, 181
    Cheesy Butternut Squash Quinoa, 164, 181
    spaghetti squash, 164
St. Germain, 198
stair-climber, 98
standing-side butt stretch, 69
staples, 186
Starbucks, 161, 162
starches, 164
step-ups, 75, 83
stevia, 166, 186
    Chia Pudding, 183
    High-Protein Frozen Banana Soft-Serve, 185
    Instant Pumpkin Pie Mousse, 184
Stewart, Martha, 212
stir-fry, 164
strawberries, 169
strength training, 12
    ball-pass crunches, 89, 94
    bent-over rows, 74, 79
    bicep curl balances, 74, 76
    body-weight tri-set, 18–28
    bosu ball push-ups with overhead press, 75,
      80–81
    chest presses on physioball, 74, 78
    dumbbell ball v-ups, 88
    dumbbell swings, 75, 82
    dumbbell v-ups, 75
    gym-based exercises, 74–95
    at home, 18–39
    inchworm triceps push-ups, 29, 30–31
    keg-stand shoulder presses, 29, 36
    kick-downs, 29, 39
    lateral pull-downs, 89, 90
    leg circles, 29, 35
    opposite-arm-and-leg supermans, 29, 38
    physioball jackknifes, 75, 86
    physioball side crunches, 75, 87
    plank, 18
    plank with single leg lifts, 29, 37
    push-ups, 18
    reverse plank, 18
    Russian twist with dumbbell, 75, 85

strength training, continued
  seated low rows, 89, 91
  side lunges, 18
  side-crunch v-sits, 29, 32
  side-plan reach throughs, 18
  single-leg deadlifts, 75, 84
  single-leg hip lifts, 18
  single-leg squat toe raises, 18
  sliding reverse lunges, 29, 33
  sliding side lunges, 29, 34
  step-ups, 75, 83
  sumo-squat shoulder presses, 89, 95
  timed body-weight workout, 29
  tricep dips with physioball, 74, 77
  triceps dips, 18
  triceps extensions, 89, 93
  walking lunges with bicep curls, 89, 92
  y supermans, 18
stress, 13
stretching, 12, 13. *See also* yoga poses
  calf foam roll, 104
  figure-four stretch, 108
  At-the-Gym Stretch Sequence, 102
  gym-based exercises, 102–109
  hamstring foam roll, 103
  hamstring stretch, 108
  hip flexor stretch, 106
  inner thigh stretch, 107
  IT band foam roll, 104
  lat foam roll, 106
  physioball chest stretch, 109
  piriformis foam roll, 103
  quadriceps foam roll, 105
  updog, 109
  upper back foam roll, 105
  Yoga Stretch at Home, 66–70
substitutes, 165–166
Subway, 162
sugar, 166
Summer Quinoa Salad, 162, 173
Summer Shandy, 197
sumo squat series, 129, 136–137
sumo-squat shoulder presses, 89, 95
Sundance Film Festival, 212
sushi, 162
Sweet Potato Fries, 164, 180
sweet potatoes, 164, 187
  Sweet Potato Fries, 164, 180
Swiss cheese, 174

T
tabouli, 162
tea, 166
teasers, 121, 127
tempeh, 161, 164
ten-minute workouts, 13, 111–151
  for arm-toning, 144
  for flat abs, 121–128
  for love handles, 138
  mountain climbers, 120
  for weight loss, 112
tequila, 198
thirty-minute Plyo-Barre cardio routine, 51–61
thyme, 181
timed body-weight workout, 29
toe touches, 121, 123
tofu, 161, 164
tomato sauce, low-sugar, 164, 187
Tone It Up 7-Day Slim Down, 193
torso-twist lunge, 69
Tosca Reno's Eat-Clean Cooler, 193
Total Body Blast, 74
toxins, 189–193
trail mix, 164
treadmills, 96
tricep dips with physioball, 77
triceps dips, 18, 25, 144, 150
triceps dips with physioball, 74
triceps extensions, 89, 93
triceps stretch, 70
tri-sets, 18–28
Tropical Green Smoothie, 161, 164, 168
tuna, 161, 162, 187
  No-Chop Healthy Tuna Salad, 172
turkey, 161, 164, 187
  Buffalo Turkey Meatloaf, 164, 182
  Low-Carb Turkey Wrap, 162, 174
twisting uprights, 41, 45
Twitter, 213, 214
tzatziki sauce, 164

U
updog, 109
upper back foam roll, 105
upright rows, 144, 149

V
Vega, 166
vegetables, 161, 164, 187
veggie burgers, 164
Virgin Diet, 190, 193
vodka, 198
  Skinny Watermelon Margarita, 198
Vodka Soda, 198

W
walking lunges with bicep curls, 89, 92
walnuts, 161, 162
  Cheesy Butternut Squash Quinoa, 181
watermelon, Skinny Watermelon Margarita, 198
weight loss, 13
  goals, 207–208
weight loss exercises
  forward leg lift toe taps, 112
  forward leg-lift toe taps, 115
  froggers, 112, 118
  happy baby dance, 112, 119
  high knees, 112, 117
  jog in place, 112, 113
  mountain climbers, 112
  reverse lunges with arm reach, 112, 114
  side lunge relevés, 112, 116
  ten-minute workouts for, 112–120
Weight Watchers, 211
weighted donkey kicks, 129, 131
Whole Foods, 166
whole wheat flour, 166
wine, 197, 198
workouts
  best time for, 209
  meals and, 157–158
wraps, 164
  Low-Carb Turkey Wrap, 162, 174

Y
y supermans, 18, 26
yoga poses
  arm circles, 70
  cat cow, 68
  chest opener, 70
  cobra, 67
  downward dog, 67, 68
  downward dog split, 67
  fold over, 67
  forward fold-over triangle, 69
  hamstring stretch, 68
  high lunge, 69
  high plank, 67
  hip flexor stretch, 68
  low lunge, 68
  low-lunge hip opener, 69
  march in place with swinging arms, 66
  mountain pose, 67
  quad stretch, 68
  standing-side butt stretch, 69
  torso-twist lunge, 69
  triceps stretch, 70
yoga stretch at home, 66–70
yogurt, Greek, 161, 164, 166
  Green Goddess Chicken Salad, 172
  Peanut Butter and Jelly Time Smoothie, 169
  Salsa Chicken Mexican Salad, 178
YouTube, 212, 213

Z
Zumba, 96